Conjuring Hope

Series: Epistemologies of Healing

General Editors: David Parkin and Elisabeth Hsu, both are at ISCA, Oxford

This series in medical anthropology will publish monographs and collected essays on indigenous (so-called traditional) medical knowledge and practice, alternative and complementary medicine, and ethnobiological studies that relate to health and illness. The emphasis of the series is on the way indigenous epistemologies inform healing, against a background of comparison with other practices, and in recognition of the fluidity between them.

Volume 1
Conjuring Hope: Magic and Healing in Contemporary Russia
Galina Lindquist

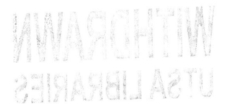

Conjuring Hope
Magic and Healing in Contemporary Russia

Galina Lindquist

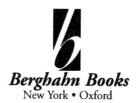

Berghahn Books
New York • Oxford

First published in 2006 by
Berghahn Books
www.berghahnbooks.com

©2006 Galina Lindquist

Paperback reprinted in 2007

Library of Congress Cataloging-in-Publication Data
Lindquist, Galina.
  Conjuring hope : magic and healing in contemporary Russia / Galina
Lindquist.
    p. cm.
  Includes bibliographical reference and index.
  ISBN 1-84545-057-4 (alk paper) -- ISBN 1-84545-093-0 (pbk)
    1. Magic--Russia. 2. Spiritual healing--Russia. 3. Russia--Religious life
and customs. 4. Russia--Social conditions. I. Title.

BF1622.R8L56 2005
133.4'3'0947--dc22

                                                                2005041135

British Library Cataloguing in Publication Data
A catalogue record for this book is available from the British Library

Printed in the United States on acid-free paper

✣ Contents

To Rita

♣ Acknowledgements

Every book emerges from a felicitous constellation of circumstances, of the intellectual, emotional and practical inputs of several people, and this one is no exception. First of all, it was made possible by a research grant from the Bank of Sweden Tercentenary Foundation (1998–0268:01), whose contribution is gratefully acknowledged. The Department of Social Anthropology at Stockholm University provided a peaceful and sympathetic environment. I am especially grateful to my colleagues Ulf Hannerz, Gudrun Dahl, Helena Wulff, Christina Garsten, Hans Hedlund, and Ulf Björklund for their encouragement, and for making day-to-day academic life easy and enjoyable.

Outside my home department, I am grateful to Pat Caplan and Kay Milton for reading and commenting on parts of the manuscript in the early stages, and to Nancy Ries for a thorough reading of the first draft. My thanks to Gasan Hage for sharing his ideas on the phenomenology of hope. I am especially grateful to Michael Jackson, who has been a source of intellectual stimulation for several years. I thank Eva Evers-Rosander for being such a wonderful friend as well as intellectual partner.

Among my Moscow colleagues, my special thanks go to my generous and caring hosts, Dr Dmitrii Funk and Dr Valentina Kharitonova from the Moscow Institute of Ethnology and Anthropology. Valentina Ivanovna Kharitonova shared with me her contacts in the world of magic, her rich research material, and her knowledge of the field of magic and healing.

My deep gratitude goes to the practitioners in the field of healing and magic. I want to mention especially Nina Georgievna Sidorchenko, whose generosity and support made both life and research easier.

I thank Don Handelman who taught me not to be afraid to be myself in thinking and writing. Many thanks go to David Budgen, whose contribution to this work goes far beyond language editing.

I thank my family for having patience with me during fieldwork and writing: my husband Anders, my sons Anton and Max, and my mother Oksana, who also provided a home for me during fieldwork. Without their support and respect this work would not have been possible.

Above all, my friend Rita was with me at every step of this project. I want to see our bond as more than our relating to one another through all those roles available to us during these years – informant and anthropologist, magus and patient, or two friends helping each other out in various circumstances. As I explain below, people tend all too easily to forget the role of their magi (and anthropologists that of their informants) when they have achieved whatever goal they had set for themselves. This is what I want to avoid, by acknowledging her share, and by dedicating this book to her.

Preface
An Encounter with 'Power'

The year was 1999 and I was in Moscow doing fieldwork. My husband and son came to Moscow to visit me; as befits foreigners on a tourist trip, we were sightseeing. An obvious sightseeing destination for any foreign tourist in Moscow is Lenin's mausoleum: a queer remnant of the epoch that, one would like to hope, is gone forever.

The long lines of Russian citizens waiting to see Lenin's body in Soviet times had now vanished. There were only a handful of foreigners waiting to pass through a cordon of militiamen, who searched their bags and checked their passports. One of them took a cursory glance at the passports of my husband and son, two Swedes with distinctly Western appearance and Swedish names, and waved them through. He dwelled, however, at length on my passport. Obviously, his eye was caught by my Russian name, and by my Russian appearance in conjunction with a non-Russian surname. The indication of Moscow as my birthplace in my Swedish passport made it clear to him that he was dealing with what in Soviet times was called a deserter, a turncoat (*perebezhchik*).

'Russian, aren't you?' he said to me with undisguised resentment. I nodded. 'Your handbag!' he bellowed. I handed him my bag, and he started to dig in it, fingering every single object. 'Here!' he exclaimed victoriously, as he extracted my mobile telephone from the bottom of it. 'Do you have a permit to carry this?' Of course I didn't. 'We'll have to confiscate your phone, and you'll have to pay a fine for breaking the rule. Hey', he nodded to his colleague, 'take her to the station.'

I shrank, remembering all the stories of harassment that befall those unlucky individuals who happen to end up in the hands of the militiamen; I thought about all the rules that I had violated without knowing it, or half knowing; about the thousands of ways militiamen had at their disposal to make my life miserable.

'And what are you doing here [in Russia at large]?' asked my interlocutor in an uninterested manner. 'I am doing research. I study magic.' 'You study magic?' he asked, and for the first time looked me straight in the eye, with keen attention. His glance was impermeable, but I met it and held it. 'Yes, I study magic', I confirmed. The other militiaman had approached and waited, listening to the conversation. The two conferred, looking again through my passport, and back at me. 'You can go', he finally said, 'But next time, remember to register your phone when you bring it in.'

This episode encapsulates several themes that are dealt with in this book. Holders of symbolic and pragmatic power do not always use it benevolently. Any inhabitant of Russia (or, for that matter, any visitor) can find herself at the mercy of powers-that-be, at a moment when she least expects it. The mechanisms through which this power works are unfathomable and murky, where a monstrous bureaucracy is enmeshed with individual inclinations and agendas and steered by emotional impulses and pragmatic considerations. Still, along with these mundane orders of power and force, there are other orders, just as tangible and significant for the native inhabitants; ones which counteract and intersect the mundane, and sometimes work minor miracles of rescue and redemption. The structures of power work through signs; these signs might be read by people differently, but they derive their pragmatic effects according to a shared logic. This logic works in ways that can also seem unfathomable, but that are all too real in their effects. As one would expect from magic, it works wonders, although in ways that can never be entirely anticipated or rationally planned.

My encounter with a representative of the law-enforcement bodies of post-communist Russia, confronted by the symbols of power partly gone, partly transformed, was an episode that belonged very much to the new times. The scenery was novel, and so was the configuration of actors; the plot, however, was strangely familiar. The militiaman and I understood each other without words, according to the formula once coined by Hannerz (to denote cultural commonality): 'I know that you know that I know' (1992). Our encounter was about complex emotions, conditioned by our respective configurations of social positioning. At first, the militiaman saw me representing all that he most deeply resented. I was one of those who had escaped the trap, avoided the hardest times, and then thought that, protected by my Swedish passport, I could come back and enjoy a bit of sightseeing, while secretly ridiculing the remnants of our past shared pride. In his readiness to show me the darker side of Russian life, there was frustration and anger. Probably, the bedrock of all this was the deep hurt his own situation caused him (his *obida* at life, an emotion that will be discussed later). His decision to let me go was partly bound up with fear: the fear of being hurt even more, of being subjected to unexpected trouble, if one messes with magic. Perhaps there was even an element of respect for someone who was not afraid to dive under the surface of mere sightseeing, to study 'these things'.

For me, this was very much like my encounter with the field of magic. It was about being exposed in a meeting face-to-face with concrete individuals, recognising the other's and one's own affects, and learning from it; about shared ways of reading signs; about gaining understanding through trying to interpret the course of events the way those involved were interpreting it. Like magic, the subject of this book, my encounter with the militia at Lenin's mausoleum was centrally about power and its social nets. Magic was a tangible force which was present in the interaction, but it was secondary to other structures, institutions and occurrences. Only by understanding all this was it possible to understand magic.

A 'halfie' in the field: studying magic in post-soviet Moscow

The problems of objectivity, reflexivity and representation connected with a peculiar situation of 'halfies' in anthropological fieldwork and writing have been discussed extensively in the last decade. Kirin Narayan (1993), for example, argued against

'... the fixity of distinction between "native" and "non-native" anthropologists, against the paradigm that emphasizes a dichotomy between outsider/insider and observer/observed.' (p. 671). Lila Abu-Lughod noted that the peculiarity of the position of 'halfies' lies 'not in any superior moral claim or advantage they might have in doing anthropology, but in the special dilemmas they face, dilemmas that reveal starkly the problems with anthropology's assumption of a fundamental distinction between self and other' (Abu-Lughod 1991: 137). What happens, she asked, when the 'other' that the anthropologist is studying is simultaneously constructed, at least partially, as self? A possible *psychological* problem, she suggested, might be the 'split of the self, ... caught at the intersection of systems of difference' (p. 140). An *epistemological* problem she indicated was the danger of excessive identification and easy slide into subjectivity.

Worries about objectivity are perhaps not as acute in today's anthropology as they were a decade ago: it has long since been realised that objectivity is never totally attainable because the outsider always stands in a definite relation with the Other due to one's specific positioning within the larger political-historical field. Nor is a fieldworking anthropologist today as keen as one probably was fifty years ago to define oneself as standing apart from the Other, at all costs. For 'halfies', I think, this separation is hardly attainable. Vieda Skultans (1998), a British anthropologist who is Latvian by birth, conveys the experience of working in her old country as unavoidably emotional. One of the feelings she describes is that of intersections of destinies, of the presupposition of a shared past that makes fieldwork encounters deeply personal. It also entails certain commitments to the people met, in practical terms when one is in the field, as well as in terms of representation when writing up. One of these commitments is to convey, as closely as possible, people's own subjectivity. As Skultans admits, it was her informants, and her wish to be true to their experience, that determined both her choice of theoretical approaches and the textual forms and strategies of her writing.

I received my training as an anthropologist in the West, but I was born and grew up in Moscow. My childhood coincided with Khrushchev's 'thaw', when memories of Stalinist terror were still fresh. My youth was the period of stagnation, and with my technical intelligentsia family background I went through a good schooling in what Oleg Kharkhordin (2000) calls dissimulation of late Soviet times: detesting the system, but being able to live in it as comfortably as your initial premises allowed. The monolith of the Soviet regime seemed eternal; the prison was a given, and people built their lives to enjoy their prison as much as they could.

I left Russia in 1986, when the Soviet system was on the verge of collapse, but had not yet actually collapsed. The processes of change, started from above in 1987, seemed no more than a ripple on the surface. The end of the 1980s was an ecstatic time, when many people in Russia were celebrating the collapse of the hated Soviet *sistema*, the colossus that many had loathed but that very few ever dreamed of so much as shaking. The beginning of the 1990s was a time of sobering-up, when many of the same people who had yesterday celebrated victory realised that they were losers. When I grew up, one of the metaphors for the Soviet system had been that of 'prison'; it conveyed the shared feeling of being subjugated, constrained and confined. A new trope that I kept hearing at the end of the 1990s was that of 'jungle'. The edifice of the 'prison' had seemed to crumble, but there were no walls nor roof to protect the dwellers from cold and rain: they were out in the wilds, and they were terrified of what was coming to replace the prison. Many people had resented and ridiculed the old home, but they knew how to live in it; suddenly, instead of that ugly, decrepit, but so livable home there was a 'jungle', and many people started to doubt their very ability to survive in it.

The thirteen years that had elapsed from the beginning of perestroika were especially devastating for two generations of Rossiiane.[1] These were my own generation, the people born in the 1950s and 1960s, and that of my parents, those born before the war and who had grown up under Stalin. Somebody had noticed that the intelligentsia of these generations were the battering-ram with which the stone gates of the old system were smashed open; they were the tool, the spearhead, that broke the seemingly unbreakable walls of the old edifice, but that was itself smashed to smithereens in the process.

The city I met was full of memories, full of shadows of the past; it was familiar, and it was at the same time utterly strange. From my earlier visits at the end of the 1980s, I remembered the mood of incredulous elation, when it was possible to say things for which one could have been imprisoned only a couple of years before; the possibility of buying in subway kiosks the books for the possession of which one could have been sent to GULAG only recently; the breathless astonishment of hearing from the media things which earlier could be only whispered in the sheltered security of one's kitchen; the feeling that the borders, which had been hermetically closed, were now wide open; the ecstatic sense of FREEDOM ...

In 1999 it was almost all gone. The spirit of the new life was conveyed by one of the many neologisms that flooded the language:

bespredel. This was a noun from the adjective *bespredel'nyi*, limitless/boundless, that in the new conditions came to connote the limitlessness of the new lawlessness, ruthlessness and cruelty that appeared to reign everywhere. It conveyed the perceived savagery of human nature that was manifesting itself relentlessly in the 'jungle', when the routines of the prison were no longer in place to put it all under lock and key. This incipient feeling of endless possibilities, of open doors and windows, of an air of freedom, was further quenched by the shock of the financial crisis of the previous year, the *defolt* of 1998. Budding faith in the new institutions of the market and banking was crushed: people lost the money they had been saving for decades, the numerous businesses that had sprung up in the preceding years went to the wall, and the tokens of plenty that started to appear on the store shelves after the emptiness of the early 1990s became unaffordable for most of the people.

Among the people I met in Moscow in 1999 – old friends and new – the intoxication of freedom had given way to a bitter hangover. A comment that I heard over and over again was that the power of ideology that had held everyone in its grip was now replaced by the power of money, less demagogic, but more conspicuous and possibly even more humiliating. Moscow appeared to me in 1999 as a city of disillusionment, resignation, even despair. The new institutions of the market and democracy, designed according to Western prototypes and apparently working well in other post-communist countries, seemed to take on quite peculiar forms in the Russia of the time. '*Demokraty*' became a derogative word, and those politicians who had been oriented towards democratic and market reforms seemed to have lost both credibility and ground with the electorate. The democratically elected Parliament, the Russian Duma, was a laughing stock amongst television viewers on account of its legislative inefficiency and its ugly brawls. It quickly became the target of bitter jokes and acrimonious accusations by the man in the street and the media alike. Business was tightly intertwined with crime, and central administration was flawed by scandals of corruption. Ethnic wars were raging in the Caucasus, echoed by terrorist and ethnic violence in the capitals. Unemployment was soaring, and the bulk of the people were impoverished. State employees, such as doctors and teachers, as well as the army of former researchers, the technical intelligentsia of the past years, and the retired and other socially vulnerable sectors of the population lived precariously, from hand to mouth, below official poverty levels, with no State-provided safety nets on which to count. The Soviet industrial colossus had almost come to a standstill; miners came from far and wide to protest on Red Square. Others were silent and tried to survive the winter by subsisting on the vegetables that they had pickled in the summer at their dachas out of town. Spectacular murders of businessmen and politicians, as well as hideous crimes of robbery and meaningless violence were much publicised in the media and brooded over by the people. The health-care system had disintegrated, good private clinics were unaffordable, and the free-of-charge alternatives were said to be staffed by money-grabbing doctors, with unhygienic wards, useless or poisonous medicines, and obsolete equipment. Moscow breathed catastrophe; it was on the brink of the unknown, in a liminal state. The old warts people had grown used to, if not fond of, were extricated painfully, without anaesthetic, and the wounds showed no signs of healing up.

Two elements of the urban landscape were most striking in their novelty, and still somehow deeply familiar in the style of their presentation. One was the explosion of erotic images, found in porn, in trashy books, videos, cheap and glossy magazines, calendars, and the like. The other was what in the West would be categorised as belonging to the market of New Age: the occult, the alternative, the paranormal, magic and healing. The erotic and the magic had always been part of people's everyday, practical life; what was new was how these phenomena, which previously used to belong to the private and the hidden, had now unabashedly come out into the open and flooded the public domain.

It was a time when a whole generation experienced something akin to nostalgia, a state of being '*à la recherche du temps perdu*', and I was no exception. I shared with many of those I met in the field the feeling of being a stranger in one's own home: ways of life we had known were gone, or had been rendered irrelevant. The brave new world was opening its hidden cellars and secret labyrinths, offering new resources. Some people grabbed and ran; others were incredulous, contemptuous, embarrassed, tempted but incapable of adapting. I shared with many the nostalgia evoked by Svetlana Boym in her 'Common Places' (1994) and analysed by Sergei Oushakine (2000) as an expression of post-Soviet aphasia, the absence of language to speak of one's experience of dissolution of one's life and self. Being a 'halfie', my fieldwork was steeped in sadness.

Being a 'halfie' also entailed a feeling of social competence that was mildly intoxicating. Writing about Soviet intelligentsia, Boym (1994) speaks about a peculiar form of communication, a sign of belonging to that imagined community, summed up in the Russian saying 'to understand each other with half-words' ('Let us understand each other with half-words', sang the famous bard Bulat Okudzhava, an idol of the intelligentsia in the 'times of stagnation'). In the late 1990s, I thought I sensed this expectation of 'shared silence, tone of voice, nuances of intonation' (ibid.: 1) among the people I met, not only those who would have counted as 'intelligentsia' proper in Soviet times, but people of different walks of life. Could it be that the trials of the 1990s had erased some demarcation lines, even as they introduced new ones? Was it because the loss of identity and direction, and the aphasic condition of numbness, the dissolution of the speaking subject (Oushakine 2000), was shared across the social groups? This was the silence that communicated, if not a shared experience, then, definitely, a shared feeling. Being a 'halfie' in Moscow in 1999, orientation in the field was easy. Russia before and after perestroika has been a complex, stratified society, where the 'native sociology' was ubiquitously present. Various groups were characterised by their own sets of dispositions and cultural designs that made it easy to recognise *svoi* (those of our own) and to categorise 'the others' with great precision. This was the essence of cultural competence that underlay discursive and performative mastery which defined the aesthetics of socialising, the joy of being together with *svoi* (known as *obchsheniie*), and also the art of manipulating the members of other social groups as resources for material favours or cultural capital. Being a 'halfie', I came inevitably to draw on this native sociology, and the knowledge that informs my analysis throughout this book is, to a large extent, my own cultural knowledge, which, I assume, I share with the people I describe.

There were, of course, pitfalls here. Often, assuming some shared tacit knowledge, people refused to answer my questions, refused to explain things I had difficulty understanding: 'How come you ask these questions? You know exactly the way these things are!' When I insisted that they should verbalise their judgements and attitudes, they often became irritated: 'Ah, you are here to study us!' As a result, I probably sometimes indulge in attributing my own analysis to people's motivations and choices. One attempt at getting around it is to keep as close as possible to people's own narratives and lines of reasoning, in what Lila Abu-Lughod (1991) called 'anthropology of the particular'.

Every time I made new acquaintances, especially in the field of magic, I took great care to announce that I was an anthropologist doing a study. This invited a specific type of exegesis. Many people were initially reluctant to look like 'pre-modern superstitious savages who believe in such things', to seem credulous idiots falling for today's modish hysteria. Their first spontaneous comments were often of a derogatory nature: 'Why this rubbish? You should look at economics instead!' Some interlocutors offered memories of their own or of their acquaintances' disappointing encounters with *ekstrasensy*,[2] impressions that more often than not were couched in terms of indignation at 'those charlatans'. When I was staying at one site trying to work closely with the practitioners, they tried to present their public façade, rendering their practice in tones of exalted praise, enumerating their spectacular successes, and favourably comparing themselves with other practitioners (whom they might also characterise as cheats or lunatics). It took time before we became close enough for me to see some of the less glamorous sides of their life.

These people, who appear in close-up portraits on later pages, did much to help me see the hidden workings of the world of magic and healing. They made a good-will gesture in allowing me to step in and to see their practice from inside. It was a gesture of trust and courage, since an impenetrable boundary of the self, an impeccable façade, is important in constructing themselves as persons of power. This presupposes that no one else has access to the weaknesses, vulnerabilities and flaws of their lives as human beings. When they admitted me that far into their lives, it was because they stopped thinking that I was there 'to study them'; because they accepted me as a friend, which meant as an equal.

Is it a breach of trust to convey the innate humanness of persons of power, to deconstruct their charisma by which I myself was often taken in? I do not know. Perhaps they would not recognise themselves in my description. Perhaps they would think that what I have to say is utterly irrelevant to the task they perceived me to have: to gain a little more understanding of the processes of transformation that they are sometimes capable of achieving through their strange gift. I could only try to capture the impressions of our meetings, and to put into words my inklings of the source of their power. Much of it had to do with the tension between the front- and the backstage of their lives, between their vulnerable insides and carefully crafted outsides – the gap crucial for their fashioning of themselves as professionals of their trade, and as charismatic individuals.

Then there were clients and patients, those on the receiver side of the channel of power. As I shall try to show later in the book, magic is a highly contested field of practice. Turning to a magus often means that a person is utterly cornered, that all else has failed and other, more conventionally acceptable channels of agency have been exhausted. Magic is stigmatised by both Church and science, and entering its terrain sometimes means that you are prepared to do something that you don't want your acquaintances, even your close friends and relatives, to know about. Therefore, personal contacts between clients and magi are an extremely sensitive matter. Turning to magi, such people expose their most painful sores, the vulnerable and probably the ugliest parts of their lives, their bitter failures, their shameful emotions and actions. Therefore, it is very unlikely that a client visiting a magus would tolerate the presence of an unknown person, least of all an anthropologist from a Western country.

I did manage to be present at some sessions, but this constituted only a small part of my fieldwork. There were two pathways to the users that gave me some understanding of the process. One was through my own friends. Hearing about the subject of my research ('What a strange thing to study! Aren't they mostly charlatans?'), and talking to me about their own problems, some of them would tentatively and with a degree of embarrassment ask me if I could recommend someone I knew, someone I thought was 'for real' or 'worthy' (*nastoiashchii* or *stoiushchii*). I usually sent them to the woman I here call Katerina, the most talented and devoted *mag* I met in the field. In return, I asked them to allow me to be present at the sessions and to tape the interaction.

As it turned out, however, making my friends the objects of study never seemed to work. First, the tape-recorder invariably failed, a fact that I could never explain in any way other than my own sloppiness, and that Katerina connected with the intentions of the higher force that was involved at all times. Second, even those of my friends who absolutely did not 'believe in these things' turned stiff when it was time for them to reveal their innermost pains, and when they faced the magus at work. My presence was clearly a disturbance, and Katerina told me so several times; I realised that this method of research was ethically problematic.

In compensation, Katerina shared with me some of her case stories. She also asked some of her patients to present to me their own narratives of how, in practical terms, magic worked for them personally; to render their versions of the stories of their collapse that had led them to her in the first place, and of the convalescence that followed. I talked to them in the kitchen of Katerina's apartment while they were waiting for their turn; or walking along to the subway station on the way home from Katerina's place; or on the telephone. Naturally, this manner of selecting the interlocutors made for bias: those who were not pleased, who thought the treatment was worthless (and there were quite a few of such people as well), did not remain as Katerina's patients, and would not want to talk to me.

Still, I met some clients whose opinions about the treatment differed from Katerina's own. There were some who thought that Katerina failed to help them, not (or not primarily) because she lacked power, but because their predicament was too difficult to be amenable to the intervention of a human being (as every magus undeniably is). There were yet others who did not perceive any betterment, and who stopped visiting her, having come to the conclusion that 'this does not work'. There was even one, referred to Katerina by myself, whom, after a month of intensive treatment, she asked to leave, and who later came to demand his money back – an unusual case, which happened to her only once or twice.

The spectacular success stories of magic came, naturally enough, from Katerina herself, as well as from a few of her faithful followers. However, my view of magic in Moscow was formed by these glowing accounts only to a certain degree. I had some friends for whom, by all accounts, Katerina's magic did definitely seem to work, when it came to comparing their life situations before and after. But, when I got back to them for their narratives, they invariably refused to talk to me about the subject. Like so many of Katerina's clients, as she bitterly commented to me more than once, when they were on the crest of a wave and no longer cornered, they tended to dismiss the impact of magic and interpret it away. When their lives picked up and they were no longer helpless, they tended to leave their magus, and chose to see their convalescence as their own achievement. They had become the agents of their own life once again, and they did not want to be reminded of anything else.

Some of these people's lives I followed during the three years that passed. For some of them, even though they refused to talk about their sensitive spots – what had led them to Katerina in the first place – I saw how their lives were changed (whether or not owing to Katerina's intervention). For others, no change was forthcoming. For some, it seemed, the magic worked somehow or other, although not quite the way they would have wanted. I discussed some cases with Katerina, and her comments also helped me understand what her magic did, and how. Being her friend for several years and having a closer insight into her life, I understood more about the charisma of the magus, the nature of her power, and its personal costs and consequences. Katerina was, unfortunately, the only practitioner with whom I remained close through these years. I lost track of the others who appear on these pages, and I have caught glimpses of their lives only accidentally, through hearsay.

People try to create their own world, to form their self and others according to their ideas of the desirable. What they end up with is the result of clashes, compromises, and concessions between selves and others, between plans and hopes and what these turn into in the real life. The resulting lived-in worlds are shaped by multiple agencies and desires, but also by what in Russia is called 'destiny' (sud'ba): by the inexorable logic of the culture and the history of the place into which they are thrown, and the world beyond.

Introduction
Post-communism and Magic in Anthropology

The 1990s have been marked by a spate of works on post-socialist countries. After the disintegration of the former Soviet Union, many Western anthropologists took the opportunity to do fieldwork in this vast and interesting, but previously closed territory. Most of them opted for remote corners of the former empire. These included Siberia and Central Asia, rural areas that had previously been out of reach (e.g. Grant 1995; Kandiyoti and Mandel 1998; Anderson 2000). Anthropologists working in urban contexts, including capital cities, have been in the minority. In their choice of subjects they concentrated on the emerging diversity of lifestyles, gender questions, youth and popular culture, on questions of memory, consumption and identity (e.g. Barker 1999; Berdahl et al. 2000). The challenge was, through detailed investigation of cultural contexts and everyday practices, to 'bridge the study of power systems and cosmologies, material practice and social meanings' (Grant and Ries 2002: ix). The present book adds to recent ethnographies, such as Ries (1997), Pesmen (2000) and Humphrey (2002), that look at modern urban contexts of post-socialist Russia, in order to explore the structures of subjectivity and personhood in addition to those of economic and social institutions. Furthermore, this book continues to uncover the 'dynamics of power in ordinary, sometimes unconceptualised and even unconscious relations, such as regarding person and the self' (Humphrey 2002: xviii). This makes it possible, burying 'ubiquitous and hoary stereotypes of "Russian culture"' (ibid.), still to understand what it means to live in a specific time and place, in a Russian metropolis at the end of the millennium. There is a fine balance between conveying this understanding and unwittingly, through anthropological writing, constructing 'a mysterious residual variable [the Russian culture], the ultimate cause of why ... people diverge from the path of development prescribed by persisting versions of "modernization theory" ' (Hann 2002: 8). However, as Humphrey suggests, 'we do not need to reify Russian culture, or any other culture, to accept that there are some combinations of previous ways, beliefs, and habits of mind' (Humphrey 2002: xxi). This book contributes to the understanding of these 'repertoires of imagination', 'habits of mind', but, also, importantly, those of heart and body. It was noted that anthropology, as well as other social sciences, 'provides us with excellent tools for describing actions, but somewhat inadequate ones for describing passions' (Perron and Fabbri, 1993: viii). This book endeavours to fill this gap, looking at emotions and passions, as they are shaped by 'habits of the mind', by the accepted patterns of language and practice, and as they are lived by the embodied socially situated subject. It is this 'grammar of affects' that shapes local cultural interpretations that frame the way people act, that determines how they interpret the actions of the others, and conceives basic social institutions. Just as, according to Humphrey's insight (2002), it is impossible to disentangle the 'economic' from the 'political', so it is impossible to disentangle the political and economic from the emotional. We need to uncover these basic patterns of subjectivity and affect if we want to understand the shape that purportedly universal institutions and ideas seem to take on Russian soil. Magic and healing, as practised in today's Russia, give an access to such understanding.

Since the birth of anthropology as a discipline, magic[3] has been 'at its epistemological centre' (Kapferer 2002: 1). In one way or another, magic seems to exist in contexts that are 'disjunctive and discontinuous' (ibid.: 14). But since magic derives its logic from the complexities of specific social practice, it can say much about these processes of rapture, the processes that can otherwise be difficult to grasp due to their chaotic and inchoate character. Another aspect of epistemological value of the studies of magic is its obvious connection with the structures of power. Magic practices thrive where power is brutal and overwhelming, where the rational channels of agency are insufficient or of limited value, and where the uncertainty of life calls for methods of existential reassurance and control that rational and technical means cannot offer. In the postcolonial, postmodern times, practices of magic reappear where they have been traditional, are reinvented where they have long since disappeared, and are constructed in new guises where traditional forms of life seem to have been eradicated by extreme social upheavals (see, e.g. Geshiere 1997).

If magic as the subject of study in anthropology has persisted through the history of the discipline, the tenor of these studies has perceptibly changed. From the classical work of Evans-Prichard (1976), where magic was seen as lying at the core of native cultural practices, to the work of Luhrmann (1989), where the magical practices of urban Westerners were presented as seemingly marginal and countercultural, the framing question being asked had always been in relation to reason and rationality. Whether seen as false science, as a mechanism for bridging social and psychological rifts, or, more recently, as a strategy of 're-enchantment' (Hammer 1997), the logic of magical thinking was to be explained with Western rationality as the baseline.

There are some recent works on magic and sorcery, however, notably those of Kapferer (1997), Stephen (1995) and Glucklich (1997), that are marked by different and novel perspectives. In these works, the ideas and instrumentalities of magic, seen as 'practices of consciousness and self' (Kapferer 1997), were conceived of as varieties of universal existential quest to secure agency and to define the boundaries of the self. Seen from these viewpoints, the analysis of magical practices served to provide insights into the deep ontologies of culture, the structuring notions that organise its workings from micro to macro levels.

Analysing the work of Mary Douglas, Kapferer notes that it opened up the exploration of magic to an anthropological understanding of social processes as formations of force and power (2002: 14). The present book is a contribution to this end, a study of the practices of power. It is not the political power of parties, governments and decrees that is at stake here. Nor is it explicitly the power of economic structures that shape and bend people's lives at the everyday level. Still, these templates of power, notably those of the market, bureaucracy and informal law-enforcement mechanisms (also known in Western parlance as 'mafia'), figure in the book as the ubiquitous background to the lives of the people who practise magic as a last resort in the hope of survival. Indeed, as I shall go on to argue in Chapter 1, the whole social field of magic and healing is enmeshed with the new market mechanisms that have changed Russia in the last fifteen years.

This book is, instead, about the power of consciousness to shape the bodies and lives of the self and others. However, the practices of magic, battles for survival in the micro domains of everyday life, are of broader interest for understanding the mechanisms at work at the macro level. This is because, as Kapferer (1997) has suggested, the powers of human intentionality, the forces of embodied consciousness, are informed by the same dynamics, and are based on the same ontologies, as those shaping politics and economics. Or, to use Bourdieu's terms (1990), diverse practices of power are informed by the same logic, on the micro and macro levels. These elusive patterns, which shape all spheres of existence for a collectivity of people sharing place and history, are not easily accessible to outside observers. Nor are they clearly conceptualised by the culture bearers themselves, at least not in everyday interactions. This is the logic of thinking, feeling and acting that endures over time, through the deepest changes in social and economic systems. It is the logic that structures the semantics of the basic linguistic terms in everyday speech, guiding the primary perception of the world, initial socialisation and everyday interaction.

This book is about the perils and wonders of intersubjectivity, and about the experience of living in the world where the conditions of being make the Western analytic term 'agency' somewhat inadequate. It is about cultural tools to change people's subjectivity in ways that makes their lives livable. It is about hope, the existential and affective counterpart of agency that replaces it where channels for agency are blocked, and presence in the world becomes precarious. This book starts from the premise, succinctly formulated by Glucklich (1997), that in the world where magic is practised, it does indeed work: when the borders of the self are blurred and permeable, human consciousness is an open system. In these cultural worlds, as Kapferer puts it (1997: 44), 'a person's existential being is inseparable from the world which is a conditionality of such a being.' When consciousness is continuous with the world, people can create and destroy this world, make and unmake each other, not only with guns and knives, but also through directed intentionality, will, passion and desire. The challenge of this study was, for me, to draw the conditions that allow for this continuity, as well as to understand *how* the practices of magic might work to change consciousness and the world; not to interpret the world I met in terms that are foreign to it, but to follow the logic of people's own interpretations. These interpretations were never made by dispassionate rational actors; instead, there were passionate players in Bourdieu's 'social games', where 'what was at stake', the *illusio*, was a matter of life and death (cf. Bourdieu 1990, 2000; Kleinman 1995). The logic of practice was inseparable from the logic of affects that shaped this practice; the rational and the emotional was continuous (see Milton 2002: 21–23).

Hope, *illusio* and 'what is at stake'

The phenomenological mode of knowledge sets out to 'bring to light the truth of experience' (Bourdieu 1990: 26). The contribution of Bourdieu, and other scholars working in the tradition of social phenomenology (most notably Arthur Kleinman and Michael Jackson) is to inquire into the conditions of possibility of this experience. They emphasise experience as an 'interpersonal medium of mediation, rather than its more usual categorization in a personal form' (Kleinman 1995: 272, n. 1). According to Kleinman, to unravel 'sociodynamics of cultural experience' (ibid.), and to understand how culture constitutes its rhythms and routines, one needs to concentrate on everyday processes and practices. What defines practices as such is the uncertainty and fuzziness resulting from the fact that they have as their principle not a set of conscious, constant rules, but practical schemes, opaque to their possessors, varying according to the logic of the situation (Bourdieu 1990: 12). The principles of practice, for Bourdieu, are to be sought in the relationship between external constraints which leave a variable margin for choice, and dispositions that are the product of historical, economic and social processes.

In his development of the theory of practice, Bourdieu has replaced the 'vacuous notion of society' (Bourdieu and Wacquant 1992: 16) by those of field and social space. Society for him is not a seamless totality integrated by systemic functions, not a common culture, criss-crossing conflicts, or overarching authority, but an ensemble of relatively autonomous spheres of 'play' that cannot be collapsed under the overall societal logic, be it of capitalism, modernity or postmodernity, nor, for that matter, socialism or post-socialism.

Bourdieu's basic notions are habitus and social field, which he also calls 'field of a game'. A field, in Bourdieu's usage, is a set of objective, historical relations between positions anchored in certain forms of power, while habitus consists of a set of historical relations 'deposited' within individual bodies, in the form of mental and corporeal schemata of perception, appreciation and action (Wacquant in Bourdie and Wacquant 1992: 16). Investment, interest, or a stake in the game is what Bourdieu calls *illusio*. It is through the notion of *illusio* that Bourdieu attempts to come to grips with the temporal dimensions of practice. *Illusio* is always oriented to the future, to something that is to be brought into being, in projects and desires, and it is therefore connected with the foundational existential condition of being, that of hope.

In a recent study where hope is made a central analytic notion, an Australian anthropologist, Ghassan Hage, admits that hope seems to be an extremely vague category, given the multitudes of feelings, discourses and practices articulated with it. Nevertheless, despite this plurality of meanings associated with hope, there is one important trait that they have in common: all of them concern the modes in which human beings relate to their future (Hage 2003: 19). According to philosopher Ernest Bloch, hope is a way in which people are determined by their future (1986: 5); as Erich Fromm puts it, hope is 'vision of present in the state of pregnancy'(1968: 13). In other words, the existential attitude of hope is the state of Being where time dimension is secured; where the present is projected into the future. This time dimension of being, the trusting expectation that tomorrow has something to offer, is a primary precondition for Being itself.

In recent anthropological writings the core phenomenological notions, those of Being and presence, are put into question. In his late work (for example, *Pascalian Meditations*, 2000) Bourdieu argued that it is not true to say that everything that people do is aimed at maximising social profit. One may say, instead, that everything that people do is to augment their social being: it is not an either/or question (epitomised by the Shakespearean 'to be or not to be') but a more or less one. Some people have more being than others, a life that is more meaningful, satisfactory, fulfilling (Hage 2003). It is the social conditions that they are thrown into that set the limits of the possible and the horizons of the desirable, even though within these conditions people are not passive recipients: they struggle, as Bourdieu puts it, to accumulate being, or, in the words of Michael Jackson, 'to transform the world into which one is thrown into a world one has a hand in making – to strike a balance between being an actor and being acted upon' (Jackson 2005: 2). Being is not a given, but an ongoing achievement, an emergent outcome of struggle, always in continual flux, waxing and waning according to a person's situation. This strive to accumulate being is what in the social science is called agency.

The notion of agency, 'the capacity to act consciously and voluntarily upon the world' (Asad 2000: 29), 'a strategic action that surmounts obstacles and transcends circumstances' (Jackson 2005: 3) has been criticised in recent anthropology. Both these writers point out that, in some societies, a person's dignity and will can be directed, not towards the transcendence of practical circumstances, but towards endurance of one's plight and 'stoic acceptance [of the fact] that one's destiny is in the hands of others' (Jackson 2005). Moreover, in some cultures agency may be located not only in the living individual, but also in the 'disembodied ancestor, household, faction, clan, [or] inter-clan alliance' (Keane 1997: 6). Agency can also be located in social institutions and other abstract entities (as in the Soviet-time slogans such as 'the Party is our steerman' (*Patriia – nash rulevoi*) or 'Lenin's cause lives and prevails' (*Delo Lenina zhivet i pobezhdaiet*); in the figures from the cultural imaginary (saints or spirits); or in inanimate objects (amulets or miracle-working icons). These cultural attributions of agency can tell us much about grids and ontologies of power in the society in question.

It appears that in the common usage of the notion of agency, understood as an instance of power with purpose and direction, two different aspects are conflated. One is the intention, desire or will to act, the other is the capacity to implement this desire or to effect this will. Obviously, there is a distinction between the will to act and the possibility to bring such a will to bear. Societies and social fields vary in terms of their enabling and constraining properties with respect to 'agency.' In addition, the social position of an individual in any society determines whether she can turn her plans into reality and construct her life more or less in accordance with her wishes (even as this same position, and the habitus that goes with it, determine the form this agency will take). For some people in certain conditions, the enabling qualities of structures are more salient that those which constrain. For others, the constraining qualities of structures are predominant. One limiting case of such constraining qualities is prison, where a person confined to its walls is more or less totally deprived of the possibility to act. Even in prison, however, a person might retain her intentionality, her desire and will to act, by designing plans for escape, for example, or by weaving internal networks of alternative power hierarchies and practices. For that to happen, this hypothetical person must have some *illusio* in the social field that her prison provides, as well as a temporal dimension to project her plans into: even in prison, one can exist if there is a hope that, for her, there is a tomorrow.

'Prison' is, historically, a well-known metaphor for Russia, as in Lenin's 'Russia is the prison of nations' ('*Rossiia – tiur'ma narodov*'), as well as in the dissident discourse of Soviet times. As already mentioned, in Russia at the end of the 1990s, the metaphor of 'prison' was replaced by that of 'jungle', or that of the 'wild' (as in the title of the book by Russian economist V.Sergeyev, '*The Wild East*', devoted to the same period). In contrast to 'prison', structures solidified to the limit, 'jungle' is another extreme, connoting the absence of structures to an extent that makes the exercise of agency difficult, rendering human beings helpless and vulnerable amidst other agencies of wild forces. If 'prison' is the accumulation of the stifling properties of structures, 'jungle' conveys the absence of its enabling properties. Both tropes reflect a situation where human existence is at the limits of survival, where there is only hope left. It is pertaining to such conditions of scarcity of resources, deprivation and structural violence, that anthropologist Enrique Rodriguez Laretta (2002) speaks about the 'precariousness of presence': a situation where we are about to lose control over our existence, at risk of being absorbed by the world. It is a condition where material channels for agency are blocked, where Being is nothing self-evident, but something one must struggle for. It is in these situations of precarious presence that people resort to other ways to secure a temporal dimension to their practices, where they can still intend, desire and wish. Hope is the existential aspect of agency, and people craft ways for themselves to secure hope even under the direst privations. One of the tasks of this book is to show how magic in Russia provides one of these ways of crafting hope.

Hage (2003) makes a distinction between subjectivity of hope, the propensity to anticipate the future even under the gravest adversities; and the 'societal hope', the capacities that societies have for the generation and distribution of social opportunities. He also notes that societies not only distribute hope unequally; they also distribute different kinds of hope. For the lack of genuine opportunities for people to make for themselves a life of dignity and fulfilment, precluded by geographical or class position, societies offer other kinds of hope. One of the examples is the promises of the Soviet slogans of the 1960s and 1970s: 'The present generation will live under Communism!' (Compare with the capacity of liberal political regimes, mentioned by Hage [ibid.] to distribute 'fantasy', a set of subliminal, and ungrounded, beliefs that individuals have a purposeful life and a meaningful future, the prospects of social mobility, manifested, for example, in so many versions of 'the American dream'.) Ideologies and religions offer the hope of salvation, which might replace the absence of the 'societal hope' of which Hage speaks, the hope of attaining a fulfilling life in this world. Millenarian hopes and fantastic dreams of quick enrichment through popular games of chance, lotteries and pyramidal schemes are characteristic of societies in poverty, insecurity and tumultuous transition. These were plentiful in Russia in the early 1990s, and they can be compared with those in Kinshasa, Zaire, as described by René Devisch. When these speculative schemes crash, 'the bitter frustration of people lead to outbreaks of sorcery accusations, as well as to pillaging and violence' (1995: 605). As Jackson (n.d.) remarks, social disintegration and misery generate obsession with chance and with violence. When the societal channels of agency are blocked, people turn to alternative ones, magic being one of them; when societal hope disappears, together with trust in electoral promises and utopian ideological projects, the culture generates alternative ways in which people can maintain their engagement with tomorrow: it offers alternative forms of hope. Criticised as 'false consciousness' that breeds passivity and futile illusions, this kind of hope still helps people survive and move on, in expectation of a better future. It allows people to retain their *illusio*, their interest and commitment to the game, to continue making stakes, and maybe, at some stations, even to win.

The metaphor of the game gives a means to take account of the element of uncertainty present in every field of human activity. Bourdieu writes that every investment, *illusio*, is associated with uncertainty, but limited and regulated uncertainty (2000: 207 *passim*). For the game to exist, the chances must be situated between subjective expectations and objective possibilities, they must be neither nil nor total. Nothing must be absolutely sure but not everything must be possible. There must be some degree of indeterminacy, contingency in the game, some 'play'. But there must also be a certain necessity in contingency, a form of reasonable anticipation. It must be provided by whatever security structures the society possesses: customary commitments or expectations that the social ties are invested with, or legal regulations safeguarding the work of institutions. The question is what happens with the game, and with the players and their *illusio*, when the social order in question shifts from orderly determination to total indetermination and unpredictability. These are the societies where the rational and legal channels of agency are blocked, deteriorated, or precluded by the designs of this society; where the 'societal hope' is scarce. Culture offers other resources, other paths for hope to take, that work according to their specific logic. This is the logic of practice that, as Boudieu put it, is not that of the logician (1990 *passim*).

Bourdieu observes that the real ambition to control the future varies with the real power to control it, which means the real grasp on the present as well (2000: 213). Those whose presence is precarious and whose future is obscure attempt to break out of the fatalistic submission to the forces of the world through acts of self-destruction: violence, terrorism, gambling, drugs, dreamlike ambitions, phantasms and uncanny imaginings. When nothing is possible, says Bourdieu, everything becomes possible, as if all types of phantasmic discourses about the future – prophesies, divinations, predictions, millenarian annunciations – have a purpose in filling up the void in what is to come, creating the nonexistent future – offering the illusory hope where the realistic one does not exist.

Bourdieu's *illusio* resonates with a key concept in the anthropology of Arthur Kleinman, who applied social phenomenology to medical anthropology in search of a language to convey the experience of suffering and pain. In his discussion of the 'professional transformations of suffering' Kleinman articulated the dissatisfaction with the interpretative project that lies at the core of classical social anthropology. He noted that the clinician 'reworks the patient's perspective into disease diagnoses and treatments that reproduce the health profession and its politico-economic sources' (Kleinman 1995: 96). But, he claims, by reformulating the patient's account of pain as moral commentary or as political performance, anthropologists participate in the same process of professional transformation of subjectivity. 'The interpretation of some person's or group's suffering as the reproduction of oppressive relationships of power or production, the symbolization of dynamic conflicts in the interior of the self, or as resistance to authority, is a transformation of everyday experience of the same order as those pathologising reconstructions within biomedicine' (ibid.). To resist the tendency towards dehumanising professional deconstruction, Kleinman proposes to draw on the 'experience-near categories', in order to understand 'what is at stake for survival, for coherence, for transcendence' (ibid.) in the daily round of happenings and transactions. That which is at stake is constrained by shared human conditions, and, at the same time, it is elaborated by the particularities of local life-worlds and individuals. 'While preservation of life, aspiration, prestige, and the like may be shared structures of relevance for human conditions across societies, that which is at stake in daily situations differs, often dramatically, owing to cultural elaborations, personal idiosyncrasy, historical particularities, and the specifics of the situation' (ibid.: 97). The central task of ethnography, argues Kleinman, should thus be not interpretation of the life of the other into the language of the self; instead, it should be to discern what is at stake for particular people in particular situations. It should mean not interpreting people, but following their own processes of interpretation along with them, making explicit the logic of practice which they follow, but of which they may not be consciously aware. It also means to try to avoid reducing people's experience of precarious presence to the 'reproduction of oppressive relationships of power or production', while attempting to uncover the grids of power in their own logic of material and semiotic practices.

One possible strategy of analysis that allows us to follow the logic of practice in its own terms, following the agents' interpretations rather than interpreting their life into an alien language, is the semiotics of Charles Sanders Peirce. The methodological strategy of elucidating the processes of metaphysical healing through the dialogue between Bourdievian social phenomenology and Peircian semiotics was brilliantly deployed in the work of Thomas Csordas (1997a,b). This approach appears fruitful to me because of its potential to grasp the interpersonal nature of human experience, and to account for its changes that are both embodied and mediated through signs. It allows one to connect changes in consciousness, mediated and expressed through signs, with those in the body and in the social situation, in individual habitus – this is what magic in Russia purports to do, and arguably sometimes does. This is because Peircian semiotics allows us to shift attention from *what* symbols mean – the task of interpretative anthropology – to *how* they mean for the people who use them, and on whom they work. Bourdieu remarks that Saussurian semiology (or, I can add, its derivatives such as structural and symbolic anthropology) emphasises that immediate understanding (and thus coherent orchestrated action according to the logic of practice) is possible only if the actors are attuned so as to associate the same meaning with the same sign, whether this be a word, a practice or a work; and the same sign with the same signifying intention (1990: 26). One of the main challenges of postmodern thought, however, was to question the shared character of this understanding, to disengage the signifier and the signified, and to see signifiers as 'free-floating' (such as, e.g. in Lash and Urry 1994). While the patterns of attribution of meaning have become increasingly individualised, however, the coherence of practices proved to be more resilient. The lesson that can be learnt from Peircian semiotics is that this shared logic of practice stems not (or not only) from the shared meaning that is associated with the same sign, but primarily from the shared ways in which this meaning is attributed: in the shared modalities of signification. No less importantly, Peircian semiotic philosophy also guides us beyond the discursive meaning, beyond the limits of symbolisation and representation, showing that many processes of signification generate bodily and emotional effects, in *presentational* rather than *representational* mode. This is where Peircian pragmaticism is tangential with Bourdieu's theory of practice: both, in their own ways, elucidate the logic of practice.

Peircian semiotics

There is a strong tradition in anthropology to use Peircian semiotics in order to account for the multiplicity of forms in which reality may be culturally imagined; and for a number of ways in which consciousness may engage with this reality, in particular in the practices of healing, magic and ritual at large. The foremost representatives of this approach are Milton Singer (1978, 1980), E.Valentine Daniel (1984), and Thomas Csordas (1997a,b). It is deep at the core of the anthropological endeavour to look for the cultural meaning, that is, to see cultural processes as a play of, or (in Daniel's expression) as a 'trafficking in', signs. Unlike the Saussurian model of sign as a signifier and a signified, and ensuing Geertzian metaphor of culture as a text to be interpreted by the observer in her own language, the Peircian model allows one to follow the agent's own interpretation. It does so by taking into account the agency of the Interpretant, the embodied consciousness on which the signs work. It also takes account of the fact that signs – objects, messages, actions – 'mean in definite ways, to someone, somewhere, and somehow' (Daniel 1984: 33).

According to Peirce, the sign consists of Object, Representamen and Interpretant. Apart from the signifier, the sign form, which Peirce calls the Representamen, and the signified, the referent, which Peirce calls the Object, he also makes reference to the Interpretant, which he defines as 'an equivalent sign, or perhaps a more developed sign' (1932: 2.228), that is created in the consciousness of the Interpreter, the person whom the Representamen addresses. Cultural analysis based on this model, as Singer (1978) pointed out, and as Daniel later reiterated, includes the empirical subject – the Interpreter on whose consciousness the signs work – as well as the empirical object – the sign form or Representamen whose referent – Object – may have a varying status in terms of veridical reality. The Objects do not have to belong to empirically verifiable reality; they can belong to cultural imaginary or, they can come to being through cultural conventions. Thus, through signification 'objects that are epistemically inaccessible' (Elgin 1996: 185) become epistemologically real – they become objects of knowledge, discourse and social life. These can be fictional, transcendental, illusive and ungraspable things, imagined sources of force and power, such as God, gods and spirits; as well as diffuse and elusive inner states of the psyche and body, as in the terms for emotions and afflictions. They have an ontogenetic quality: by entering into the semiosis of social life, they act upon people and generate new realities. Examples are spiritual beings who become social persons in traditional cultures; characters of the religious imaginary, like Our Lady and saints, who are present in the lives of faithful Christians of certain denominations; or imaginary characters created by fiction and media, as is the case in the West. All these, present as social persons, can have very real effects on their human consociates, by healing or hurting them, by causing fear or love. Social actualities, such as institutions, facts and events, as manifestations or vessels of meaning, are Interpretants of some earlier semiotic chains. They can well be considered as socially and existentially real without the need to accrue such an ontological reality to their original generative Objects. One obvious example of this is the Christian Church. As a complex of social institutions, it is a real social fact that has emerged, and continues to develop, from one single Object, the person of Christ, whose ontological reality one may or may not accept.

The mechanisms of signification are further illuminated by applying the Peircian categories of *how* the signs signify. According to their modes of signification, Peirce distinguishes between Icon, Index and Symbol. Icons signify, as Pierce puts it, 'by community in some quality', be it in appearance (outward resemblance), in inner structure, or in function. A portrait painted in the style of realism, as well as a photographic portrait, are iconic Representamina of their Objects, the persons who sat for them. The 'similarity in appearance' evidenced in portraits and in photos is the most obvious and most often quoted criterion of iconicity. A chemical formula is an icon of a chemical compound, due to similarity in inner structure (which may be confirmed, say, by pictures taken under the electron microscope). A solarium apparatus can be regarded as an icon of the sun, through the 'similarity of function' (see Eco 1986).

Indexes signify by reference, like demonstrative pronouns and prepositions, and also by 'existential relation' that can be factual contiguity or pragmatic causality. So, a photograph is an index of its Object, since this Object is a direct cause of the chemical and physical processes (refraction of light and chemical reactions) that in the end result in a photographic image. The Shroud of Turin is seen by the faithful as an indexical sign of Christ. Traces in the sand are indexes of a person who has walked there; clouds in the sky are indexes of coming rain; concerted actions of a group of soldiers are an index of an order of their commander to take up arms. The qualities of iconicity and indexicality coexist in many signs, as, for example, in metonymic representations. A lock of hair is an indexical sign of the person to whom it had belonged, having once been 'part of the whole' (and thus in an existential connection with it); it is an icon because it shares its inner structure. Without going further into this subject, let me point to the obvious affective charge of such representations: the Shroud of Turin, as well as the lock of hair of someone loved, convey the immediacy of the living presence of the Object and can thus affect the Interpreter on a deeper emotional level of that cognitive deciphering than the interpretation of symbols might involve.

Finally, symbols signify by convention, and this is the type of signification that has been afforded greatest attention in most analyses of representation. The interpretation of symbols within a culture is made on the basis of the existent agreements between indigenous Interpreters, who have knowledge of the shared Ground. But convention, cultural knowledge, or habit of interpretation, might also determine the indexical and iconic modalities of signification. While the connection between the wind and the weather-cock, or the feet and the traces in the sand (textbook examples of indexes) are of a physical nature, that between the order to take up arms and the subsequent actions of a group of people is based on cultural conventions, although the mode of signification is clearly indexical. Likewise, the Shroud of Turin indexically signifies the suffering of Christ only for the faithful who know the New Testament story. Since power implies, among other things, a potential for transformation of state, signs of power signify indexically – a point made central in the magnum opus of Roy Rappaport (1999) that I shall return to below. But it is the shared cultural knowledge of Interpreters about the symbolism of power that gives these signs their indexical potency: the agreement between the soldiers that they are to obey their officer (as at the order to take up arms), or that between the drivers in the streets of Moscow that a certain sign of a traffic police means that they have to stop (and pay the bribe in order to be able to drive further). The domain of semiosis that involves changes of state under the impact of signs conceived as icons and indexes through cultural convention is closely connected to cultural conceptualisations of power and force, and will be one of the main themes of this study.

As Daniel (1984) notes, every cultural system is a panoply of iconic, indexical and symbolic signs, and it is the culture that decides *how* these signs mean to its bearers. There is a rich anthropological tradition of studying the polysemic character of signs, or the multivocality of symbols: cultural conventions on meaning are far from clearly defined, and even where they are, there are always countercultural discourses that offer their own, differing or dissident, meanings of symbols. Daniel shifts the attention 'from polysemy or multivocality to polychromy or multimodality' (ibid.: 39). Signs that have conventional meanings can conceal within them iconic and indexical aspects. Symbolic aspects of some signs, especially nonlinguistic sings, like graphic images and gestures, or other movements, are minimised or nonexistent; these signs signify only in iconic and indexical ways. Culture dictates which facets of signification are more important in a particular instance, and cultural knowledge implies competence in what modes of signification are implied: *how* signs signify.

Further, different cultures valorise, and emphasise, some modes of signification over others. Daniel notes that in Western culture, the symbolic mode of signification is predominant, whereas in South Asia iconicity is valued over symbolisation. In Russia, the iconic mode of signification is important, not least where power is concerned in all its guises. More generally, Rappaport (1999) argues that in rituals, especially those invoking the power of the ineffable, the divine and the sacred, iconic and indexical modes of signification become of primary importance. If we consider magic and healing to be a specific instance of the invocation of the Divine, the embodiment of an ineffable but potent agency, then it is no wonder that both iconic and indexical modes, or, as Taussig (1993) puts it, Copy and Contact, are crucial in magic and healing. In Russia as elsewhere, photographs, effigies such as wax dolls (copies/icons), personal things such as handkerchiefs (indexes of the Object, since they have been in contact with her), and especially body materials such as nails, hair and blood (both icons and indexes) are considered the best substrates on which to work the most powerful magic. This has been discussed by many scholars of the subject, from Frazer (1922) through Mauss (1972), to Evans-Prichard (1976) and Tambiah (1990). Sympathetic and homeopathic magic works on the principles 'a part for the whole' and 'like treats like' (both these modes of relatedness involve an existential or causal relation, i.e. indexicality, and a community in some quality, i.e. iconicity). The point that should be emphasised here is that it is culture that designs and determines the modes of signification: the knowledge of *how* signs signify is a cultural knowledge, a part of being in the world in a certain way, and they exert their effects in ways that are culturally envisioned. Cultural conventions of signification are indeed what makes some signs work as icons and indexes. It is the Interpreters' awareness of indexical and iconic modes of signification that constitutes their efficacy, and grounds their pragmatic consequences.

Power

There are few concepts that have preoccupied Western thought in the last millennium as much as the concept of power. Michel Foucault, who did much to unravel the workings of power, also recognised how difficult it is to grasp it. One of his many takes on power was to see it as 'an open, more or less coordinated ... cluster of relations'. The problem posed by Foucault in this instance was to provide ourselves with a grid which makes possible an analysis of these relations (Foucault 1980: 199). One way of applying Foucault's approach is to forego the question what power *is*, and to see what it *does*, and in what domains of social life, and in what types of relations, it manifests itself.

A good minimal definition, admittedly modest, but all the more applicable to the analysis of everyday practice, has been suggested by anthropologist Andre Droogers (1994): 'Power is the ability to get things done.' If power is the way of getting things done, then the ways people see things get done are what Foucault calls a grid for the analytic relations of power. What is at issue here are the indigenous ontologies of power: how people conceptualise causality and the driving force of transformations and how they relate to their own ability (or inability) to act and counteract. The indigenous mechanisms of signification are crucial here. Anthropologists studying ritual and religious expressions, notably Roy Rappaport (1999) and Thomas Csordas (1997a), demonstrated that iconic and indexical modes of signification are at the core of the workings of power. The culture bearers usually know no more than the analysts about what power *is*: its sources, or, as Foucault puts it, its genesis is obscure for those on whom it works (perhaps this very obscurity is a *sine qua non* of its existence).

17

But people know power when it acts on them. They know it indexically, through its results; and they also recognise power in its instances, or, in semiotic terms, in its icons. Power is often presented iconically and it acts, and is interpreted, indexically. Through these modes of semiotic mediation power becomes objectified, and made real as a lived force; recognised and accepted through the shared modes of signification, it achieves its transforming effects. One of the main themes of this book is the unravelling of the significations of power. Using the notion of the 'icon of power' I try to discern the ways in which agency is conceived, attributed and recognised, thus being taken to act indexically, sometimes with real effects. These effects, I argue, are also constructed indexically, when the power of charismatic individuals triggers the agency of the clients. If this power cannot change the material channels that potentiate the structural dimension of agency, it can blow life in its affective dimension: to awaken hope.

The self

If magic is an instantiation of power, a culturally conceived mode of action, then the object of this action, as well as the acting subject, is the self. When Michele Stephen wrote her 'A'aisa's Gift' (1995), the juxtaposition of magic and the self had an odd ring: magic was a traditional subject of anthropological study, while self as an object of analysis was extolled as one of the themes of new anthropology. Now, almost a decade later, after the spate of works on self and person, the attention to self as a locus of culture seems almost conventional. Still, even now self is a problematic notion, primarily because, being rooted in the English language as an accepted, self-explanatory analytic term, it lacks equivalents in many other languages. As early as 1992, Whittaker made an overview of different definitions of the term 'Self' as used in recent anthropological debate, and of different meanings and intentions that these definitions might serve. At one conceptual pole, there are phenomenological approaches that seek to reconstruct individual self-awareness as a unique, particularistic, experience of being human, both connected to, and separated from, others. At the other pole, there are cultural templates of the self; the self as objectified by culture, whether the latter is understood in an interactionist, symbolic or normative sense. Of course, the cultural-constructivist and the experiential aspects of the self are interconnected and mutually illuminating: one experiences oneself as a more or less individuated entity, both separated from, and connected to, others, through the modes of perception and plays of signification provided by culture, which also provides definitions of social codes through which this bonding and separation are effected.

A concept of 'self' that could be useful for anthropological analysis should capture this interconnectedness of individuation and separation, and the dynamic character of embodied consciousness as a play of signs, without reifying the bounded atomistic 'self' intrinsic to the Western ontology of the person. The definition of the self proposed by Csordas in 1997b goes a long way in capturing these dynamics of interconnectedness of various aspects, without conflating the Western folk model with the analytic term that could be applicable in various contexts. Csordas defines 'self' as the indeterminate capacity to participate in the on-going process of orientation and engagement in the world. Two basic traits that, according to Csordas, characterise this process are effort and reflexivity. They are connected with the two sides of consciousness conceived semiotically as a play of signs. The former is the embodiment, and the sheer resistance of the material and social structures of the lived-in world that the human being has to navigate in order to survive. The latter is awareness, the ongoing conceptualisation of the world by the individual through implicit cultural ontologies, as well as through more explicit cultural codes and rules. They are also connected with two sometimes conflicting directionalities of the self: towards autonomy and individuation, through consolidation of the boundaries of the self; and towards the creation of social bonds that reflect the self and provide the terms for identity and belonging. The human being everywhere strives to be both bonded with others and to be individuated. Bonding and individuation are two opposite existential directions that need to be constantly monitored through effort and reflexivity.

In his brilliant recent work on practices of self-fashioning in Soviet Russia, sociologist Oleg Kharkhordin (1999) showed how the Soviet ideological project led to the development of a particular kind of the self – both collectivist and individualistic, forged in cruel pedagogical practices and the stale rituals of officialdom, but also in tightly knit informal groups of friends. A striking feature of the Soviet self, argues

Kharkhordin, was its dependence on the social groups in which it belonged. The individuality of a Soviet person was always and only 'a corollary of mass-production'. It existed only insofar as the person was included in the network of social relations (p. 195), and it was built with the symbols of identity, values and ideas that these relations provided. This being so, the state of 'post-Soviet aphasia' (the loss of language) discussed by Oushakine (2000) comes as no surprise. With most of the formal and informal groups – *kollektivy* – gone or transformed, there is no symbolic language to define the self, 'no cues about the direction to follow, no channels for one's identificatory process' (p. 995). As the respondents in Oushakine's study say, 'a post-Soviet person is one who is lost in the world, one who tries [and is unable to] to find her self ... [one who is] totally naked – spiritually, materially and nationally' (ibid.). One of the reasons for this aphasia, according to Oushakine, is the absence of the legitimate, emotionally and cognitively acceptable 'fields of cultural production'. The challenge of this book will be to show how magic can provide an alternative, albeit home-grown and transitory, to those disappearing fields, thus giving hope for the self to be reassembled and redefined.

Belonging and individuation, bonds and autonomy are two push-and-pull modes of being-in-the-world of which magic is only one instance. As several students of magic have noted (e.g. Stephen 1995; Glucklich 1997), magic thrives where human bonds are strong, and where the boundaries of the self are permeable and fuzzy. But, as Stephen in particular aptly demonstrated, magic can also be seen as a striving to solidify the borders of the self, to effectuate individuation, and to diminish the effects of those bonds that define the social contours of the self and provide the terms for its reflexivity (defining the social others through which the self conceives of itself). As we shall see, the making and unmaking of one's own and other selves through the manipulation of the boundaries and the bonds that define it are at the very core of magic in Russia. Manipulation of the boundaries of the self, their consolidation beyond what is accepted in a particular culture is what underlies personal charisma, the power that some individuals accrue to become professional practitioners.

These social and structural aspects of the self, however, are only part of the story. The other part consists of passions, the elusive substance of subjectivity, much more difficult to grapple with using the tools of social sciences. Scholars agree that emotions play a central role in structuring our sense of the self (see, e.g. Lupton 1998 for an overview of the work on 'emotional self'). As Michele Stephen puts it, self is constituted of feelings and desires – affects – directed towards the world and the other people in it (1995). It will be argued that the practices of magic alter self and subjectivity by manipulating affects and changing subjectivity, ultimately by augmenting its temporal dimension, the dimension of hope. In Greimas's lexicon of affects (Greimas and Fontanille 1993) hope is defined as desire + time + uncertainty. When uncertainty becomes too high (in Bourdieu's terms, when the gap between the *illusio*, the stake in the game, and *lusiones*, the chances to win, is too great), the time dimension is warped, and hope cannot sustain the player anymore. Magic deals with uncertainty (cf. Whyte 1998), neutralising its destructive potential, and making hope, as a mode of existential orientation, once again possible.

Thus, the main challenge of this book is to bring together structural and passional dimensions in understanding transformations of the self in a specific cultural context. The study of magic is particularly suitable for this purpose. This is because, as Bourdieu noted, the logic of magic is deeply connected with the experience of emotions and passions (1990: 93). But, he continued,

> to understand magic means more than reconstituting its internal logic. It also means restoring its practical necessity by relating it to the real conditions of its genesis, that is, to the conditions in which both the functions it fulfils and the means it uses to its ends are defined. It means describing brutally material basis of the investment in magic [...] which causes the life dominated with anxiety about the matters of life and death to be lived as an uncertain struggle against uncertainty. It means trying to name, even if one cannot really hope to make it felt, this collective experience of powerlessness which is at the basis of a whole view of the world and the future. (1990: 97)

I would add that to understand magic in Russia means to understand the ways cultural creativity provides people with their share of what Bourdieu calls *conatus*, augmentation of being: in the conditions of precarious presence, to evoke the future to live for, and to give them strength to make a stride into this future.

Notes

1. The term was coined during perestroika in the spirit of local political correctness, and it has been used since instead of 'Russians' (*russkiie*) to embrace the totality of Russian as well as non-Russian groups living in the Russian Federation. See Balzer (1999), Humphrey (2002).
2. *Ekstrasens* is a popular term for people who supposedly possess paranormal abilities. It comes from 'extra-sensorial perception', the ability to perceive that is above the usual human five senses.
3. Authors recently writing on the subject question the use of Western categories such as 'magic' and 'sorcery' in describing indigenous practices. These terms, the critics argue, bear connotations of arrogance and contempt, inherited from the founding fathers who saw magic as 'bastard science' and 'corrupt religion' (for an excellent discussion, see Tambiah 1990). Another objection to these labels is that they artificially group together a highly diverse set of practices that may not be reducible to one term (Kapferer 1997). The tendency thus has been to abandon these terms and to use the indigenous labels instead. In my own case, the choice is simple. The set of practices that strive to change matter through mind is in Russian called *magiia*, and its practitioners are known as *magi* (sing. *mag*).

Chapter 1
Marketing Magic

While the occult, by definition, is a hidden knowledge, urban magic in big cities is a conspicuously public phenomenon. As such, it is created by the media and upheld by the market as a thriving field of service and commodity exchange. The upsurge of paranormal performances and services in Russia in the late 1990s subsided somewhat by the beginning of the 2000s. By then, magic and healing came to occupy a more stable place on the market of services, at times converging with more conventional kinds of interpersonal help, such as business consulting, psychotherapy, and various types of health care.

According to the estimates of Russian sociologists, in 1998 there were more than 50,000 officially registered 'specialists in non-traditional[1] healing methods' in Moscow alone (Pachenkov 2001). For the whole of Russia, *Nezavisimaia gazeta* (10.06.1996) gave an approximate number of 'hundreds of thousands of "magi, sorcerers and fortune-tellers" [*magi, kolduny, predskazateli*]'. This figure seems to me rather arbitrary, since there are plenty of practitioners who never register nor advertise; there are also people who practise magic and healing in their free time, treating friends and relatives, and combining these activities with other professions that may have nothing to do with either medicine or magic. Thus, an informant told me about a female lawyer who held an administrative job at a ministry in Moscow, while also practising massage, bone-setting and hand-healing in the evenings; he referred to her healing as highly efficient.

The question that concerns me in this chapter is the seeming contradiction between the occult character of magical knowledge, and its spread and visibility as a social and economic field in post-perestroika urban Russia. As a segment of the market of goods and services, magic offers alternative means to earn a living to those who could have become victims of the post-socialist transformations.

Russian sociologist Oleg Pachenkov (2001), who studied the market of magic in St Petersburg, formulates the same paradox in Weberian terms: he asks how the 'irrational' world-view on which magic practices seem to be based is compatible with the very rational methods of marketing and advertising that its proponents employ. As providers of goods and services, magi and healers operate in the conditions of tough competition, and to market their services they must deploy the strategies that work for other kinds of business as well. It may be suggested, however, that the very dissemination of a magical world-view may be seen as a consequence of market mechanisms at work: the ideas on which magic rests are made public through media channels that are the new infrastructures of business and marketing.

This said, it must be added that magic is not like any other sphere of business activity: even though its cultural roots are deep, its legitimacy is utterly contested. The strategies of legitimation that I shall trace in the texts of advertisements are parallel to marketing strategies that are singled out by Pachenkov. However, as I shall try to show, there is more at stake in this self-presentation than mere marketing. What practitioners try to secure is not simply a business niche; they also try to carve out for themselves an acceptable social identity and a worthy place in the moral domain. The strategies of legitimation that are used to these ends are indispensable for practitioners' self-construction as attractive and desirable, as charismatic individuals, which, as will be argued later, is the main precondition of the effectiveness of their healing.

Magic in Russia as a public field

The magic and healing services are broadly advertised in several specialised newspapers. The number of these newspapers varies depending on the financial conditions of the publishers – two or three such newspapers disappeared after the economic crash of 17 August 1998, the black day for Russian entrepreneurs and the incipient middle class. Other similar newspapers, such as *Oracle* and *Hidden Power* (*Tainaia vlast'*) survived the crisis and circulate in millions of copies, and in addition new ones crop up. These newspapers are a source of information about rediscovered and reinvented folk beliefs and practices, providing advice as to how to behave during fasts or how to use cards or coffee grounds to predict

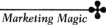

the future or to find a loved one. They also feature articles on the era of Aquarius (known as New Age in the West), astrology, the magic of numbers and names, paranormal and occult phenomena in everyday life, advice on how to acquire inner harmony, outer beauty and material wealth. In much of their content these newspapers recall the same genre in the West, the New Age discourse.

While in the West similar newspapers would advertise courses on inner development, shamanism and crystal healing, Russian newspapers give their pages over to advertisements for magical and healing services offered by diverse specialists. These professional magi and healers might work individually in rented premises or in private homes. Alternatively, they might receive clients in so-called 'centres', establishments where several magi work together in a more institutionalised setting.

The field of magic in Russia can be distinguished analytically from that of healing, even though in real life this distinction is often blurred. Healers claim to treat physical health problems and receive patients in clinic-like parlours complete with diagnostic equipment. Such healing clinics offer a complex range of services, including massage, bone-setting, acupuncture, homeopathy and herb medicine, in addition to the laying-on of hands. The latter is known in Russia as 'bio-field healing', but is sometimes also referred to as extra-sensorics[2], bio-energo-therapy, enio-therapy (*enio* – the abbreviation for *energo-informatsionnyi obmen* – means 'energy-information exchange'), etc.

The scope of diseases that healers promise to cure is indeed vast. Below is the list of disorders mentioned in the newspaper advertisement of a healing centre where I carried out participant observation. 'Diseases of the gastro-intestinal tract: gastritis, cholecystitis, colitis, stomach ulcers, enuresis, impotence, enteritis, haemorrhoids; Gynecological and urological diseases: nephritis, cystitis, kidney stones; diseases of the endocrinal system, bone diseases, arthritis, ostheochondrosis; restoration of hearing and vision. Skin diseases such as psoriasis, eczemas and rashes. Diseases of the reproductive system; infertility, impotence; delayed development and neurocerebral paralysis in children.' (newspaper advertisement for Nina-S, 1998). Some healers even claim to remove benign tumours such as myomas and adenomas, and also provide general rehabilitation after major surgery and hospital treatment, after heart attacks and strokes. It is easier to say what they do not treat, or at least are always reluctant to treat, or for what they do not promise any results. One such disease is cancer, another is schizophrenia together with other kinds of grave mental disturbances.

Crucially, to open a clinic, a healer must have a medical degree. Many practitioners do have so-called vocational training in nursing schools and specialised medical schools, and some also have degrees from prestigious medical colleges (it should be noted in parenthesis that buying such a degree in Russia is a matter requiring only a little additional effort). Whether their medical diploma is real or bought, healers who work in such healing centres are, by and large, people with biomedical knowledge on the level of a medical professional. Biomedical education leaves many healers equipped not only with a 'scientific' paradigm, but also with a good working knowledge of anatomy, pathology and pharmacology. Therefore, they are familiar with medical terminology, so that their diagnoses are presented to patients in conventional biomedical language, in line with (confirming or modifying) those obtained in regular health-care institutions. Such healers need the diagnostic equipment to 'objectively' assess, and to have patients witness with their own eyes the results of their healing, when a tumour, for example, gets smaller or disappears from the ultrasound picture.

While healers who work in clinic-like establishments tend to have some background in health care, magi come from a wide variety of groups that span the entire social spectrum. Among full-time or part-time practitioners I knew, or heard about, in Moscow, there was an accountant, an architect, a bank teller, a kindergarten teacher, a housewife, a factory worker and a shop clerk. The rule of thumb is that magi tend to have permanent clients from the same social stratum, although a mark of a good magus is that he or she can efficiently interact with clients across social borders.

Unlike healers, who define both ailments and treatment in biomedical language, magi cater for social, emotional and psychological problems, those of love and family, alcohol and drug addiction. In addition, many magi offer to handle the issues of jobs and business, acting as business consultants or security advisers (for more on business magic in Russia, see Chapter 7, this volume; Lindquist 2000b, 2002a; and Pachenkov 2001).[3]

While healers present their interventions in purely medical-scientific terms, deritualising their actions to the greatest possible degree, magi deal with the same ontological disturbances in a more ritualised way. The stock of ritual means is idiosyncratic to individual magi, and they are allowed, indeed expected, to display a good deal of personal inventiveness. In Russia, as elsewhere, people tend to distinguish between black and white magic. The former is understood to harm, the latter, to do good. Definitions of good belong to the moral domains of culture; but also, to varying degrees, they are wilfully conceived by individuals, in terms of their perceived understandings of what is fair and just in the contexts of their own lives.

In Soviet times, the moral domain was a muddled ground, since 'The Moral Code of the Builder of Communism', as Soviet ideologists referred to morality, was perhaps never taken seriously by the vast majority. Post-perestroika, questions of morality are still being sorted out. The Church is called on to bring clarity to this area, but its teachings do not always sit easily with folk models of morality. For example, in the popular understanding, to bring an errant husband back into the family fold is a moral deed, and to punish the mischief-maker, as well as his promiscuous seducer (a paradigmatic act of black magic), will not necessarily be seen as reprehensible. Russian folk magic has a range of spells and rituals intended to effect punishment and retribution, for example to render 'the shameless he-goat' (*kozel besstyzhii*) impotent with respect to all other women but his own wife. This measure would certainly be considered an act of black magic by the husband and his mistress, while the wife would regard it as a morally defensible act aimed at strengthening the family and restoring a just social order.

Since in human life good and bad are hopelessly entangled, in the popular understanding the distinction between black and white magic tends to be made in terms of efficacy. The results of 'white magic' are tacitly expected to be limited by God's will: the client must accept that if it is not His will, the straying husband will not come back and the son will not be cured of his alcohol addiction. In contrast, black magic is presented by its practitioners as being highly effective. In advertisements, the self-designated 'black magi' often promise 'a 100 percent result guaranteed or money back'. Significantly, these 'black magi' often flaunt the fact that they charge high fees, and claim as their sources Haitian voodoo, Brazilian condomblé, Celtic druidism, or Scandinavian rune magic. This connection in the popular imagination between money, potency, otherness/the foreign, and evil/the Devil is far from unique to Russia (see, for example, Taussig 1987).

As far as white magic is concerned, the so-called 'folk magic' is based on traditional folk spells and ritual actions, taken by the magi from numerous old and modern, popular and scientific books on Russian folklore. The female magi who practise folk magic call themselves *babki* or *babushki*. While *bábushka* is the Russian for grandmother (a kinship term), *babka* (and *babuska* as well) is also a popular term for the old wise women who have always operated in Russian villages, healing humans and cattle and offering magical services to neighbours for a small fee. Modern urban *babki* can present themselves as wise old women with a veneer of village homeliness and a simple and familial charm (such as baba Niura, also known as *Anna-spasitel'nitsa*, Anna the Saviouress, mentioned in Pachenkov 2001). But they can also be elegant and successful young women, like a personage who calls herself *'babka* Malan'ia' whom I briefly met in Moscow. The latter received clients in an up-to-date office with a guard at the door, video-screens and a secretary typing away at a computer. *Babka* Malan'ia (and a number of people like her) was in the 1990s a frequent guest on television talk shows, where she offered expositions of the folk healing tradition in an elegant wrapping palatable for urban television viewers. This appearance in the media can be considered as another marketing strategy or advertisement channel; but it is also a means of disseminating and 'normalising' a world-view that, for the young urban intelligentsia, can still seem unusual, unfamiliar and 'irrational'.

Understandably, magi who have become public personalities can hardly work alone: on the material on St Petersburg, Pachenkov talks about what he calls 'entrepreneurial teams'. Such teams, he writes, can comprise the *babushka* herself; her assistant(s) who deal with what in Russian is called *'piar'* (coming from PR, or public relations): journalists, clients, law enforcement authorities, etc.; a business director who deals with the financial side, as well as for the marketing and advertisement campaigns to launch the magus as such – the process known in contemporary Russian as *raskrutka*, literally meaning unleashing or spinning up; and the service personnel such as permanent guards and cleaning ladies (Pachenkov 2001: 106). These 'village wizards' are thus very much unlike their rural counterparts evoked by the term *'babka'* in popular imagination.

Taking the name of *babka*, the modern practitioners position themselves both on the market and in the moral domain, subscribing to a certain strategy of legitimation, as detailed below.

Other magi who do not claim to have village roots, like my friend Katerina, may still make extensive use of the literature on folk spells and rituals. In addition they may also have read Alice Bailey, Aleister Crowley, Aliphas Levy, Henry Papus, and other Western sources of magic, which are abundantly available in translation at Russian bookstores.

Most of the rituals performed by 'white magi' are variations on a few specific themes, and these themes lean heavily on church attributes and paraphernalia. Many magi, both those who claim folk or rural descent, and those of the more syncretistic brand, consider themselves pious Russian Orthodox Christians. They go to church regularly, follow church holidays and prescriptions, fast according to the elaborate Orthodox schedule, wear a cross, surround themselves with church candles and icons, regularly acquire water blessed in the church, and make plentiful use of church paraphernalia in their rituals. As a standard part of their treatment of all kinds of complaints, many magi ask their patients to buy a popular brand of mineral water called 'Holy Spring' (*Svyatoi istochnik*) bottled by the Church as a part of its thriving business activities, and blessed by the Patriarch himself (as the bottle label informs the buyer). The magus then charges the water with her own energy and instructs the patient to drink it at certain times of the day, and to wash their hands and face with it. Magi also often serve as church missionaries in their dealings with clients, as many of them prescribe as part of their treatment to go to confession and Communion, to buy tapers and icons, to make a pilgrimage to some holy place, to be baptised if they have not been so, or simply to go to church for a liturgy, a prayer, or the blessing of water.

The Russian Orthodox Church has become a major source of moral guidance and authority in Russia, and magi are not the only people who look towards the Church in their attempts to forge legitimacy for their activities. In her article on home birth in contemporary Russia, anthropologist Ekaterina Belousova (2002) describes transformations in the rhetoric and ideological moorings among the Russian home birth movement. In the end of the 1980s their proponents presented themselves in broad terms of 'basic spirituality', familiar from the New Age paradigm, blending Russian Orthodox elements with those of

Yoga, Zen Buddhism and transpersonal psychology. In the end of the 1990s, however, the ideologists of the movement were talking about the dangers of 'alien' practices, casting it, instead, in the idiom of 'Russian Orthodox mentality'. The midwives' use of traditional folk remedies and other elements of folk magic presented for them no contradiction with their Russian Orthodox identity. Just like other areas of health-care practices that reemerged alongside the bio-medical ones, home birth had to latch on to the Russian Orthodox Church to wield legitimacy. Later in this book we shall see how clients of magi use the symbols from the Russian Orthodox repertoire to express the perceived positive changes in their lives and selves. While in the case of home birth this reference seems innocuous, the Church itself having no ideological objections to the practice per se, for magi (and their clients) this reliance on the Church can be rather dubious. The Russian Orthodox Church is one single most fierce opponent of all sorts of healing and magic, especially of those couched in terms of 'spirituality' rather than 'science'. Ironically, one of the very few sociological analyses of magic and New Age movements in the Russian-language literature is offered by a Church ideologue, Deacon Andrei Kuraiev, who denounces all varieties of what he calls 'Occultism in Russian Orthodoxy' (1998).

The roots of contemporary magic

Magic and healing, which became conspicuous after perestroika, did not spring from nowhere. Strands of magic and healing found in today's Russia find meaning and legitimacy in the corresponding sociocultural domains of the past. In Communist Russia official ideology strove to dominate all spheres of life, including, not least, the health-care system. The only officially allowed, and bureaucratically established, type of health care in the Soviet era was biomedicine. This comprised a well-established network of outpatient clinics, primary maternal and child care, and a vast number of pharmacies selling a large variety of prescription drugs and medicines over the counter. Clinics and hospitals were free of charge, and backed up by a solid system of laboratory research.

This does not mean, however, that there was no de facto medical pluralism even during Soviet times. On the contrary, what was broadly termed 'alternative medicine' was developed semi-underground, and used, by choice or necessity, or by way of experiment, by people from different walks of life. These 'alternative' methods were all the more popular since they had an aura of being officially stigmatised, if not outright forbidden.

As an illustration, let me relate an episode from my own past. I grew up in a family belonging to the technical intelligentsia – atheists, with no roots in the village. There were no special health problems in the family, and current ailments were dealt with by heart drops, antibiotics and bactericide drugs that were part of every home pharmacy. When my son was three months old, in 1979, he suddenly developed a bad case of inguinal hernia. For such an emergency, the regular institutions of local, outpatient and primary childcare were clearly insufficient and a high-powered child surgeon, found through personal connections, was duly contacted. One of his references was that he had undergone advanced training in France, and that he spent part of his time there, working in a big Paris hospital. For a private consultation fee of 60 roubles (half of a month's salary), the surgeon examined the baby and gave his verdict. This type of hernia, he said, could be removed only by surgical intervention; in rare cases it disappears by itself in girls, but never in boys. But the baby was too small for surgery. We were to wait three months, and then the surgeon undertook to do the job himself. He said that this type of illness was not directly life-threatening; but the baby should not be allowed to cry loudly, in order not to strain the groin muscles. This was more easily said than done, as the boy was obviously in pain and screamed continuously. His paternal grandmother, who lived on one of the new residential estates in the outskirts of Moscow, suggested consulting a neighbourhood healer ('*babka*'), who, luckily, was well known for being a specialist in treating hernias. When I mentioned this therapeutic option to my parents, they were indignant: surely I was out of my mind, to fall prey to silly superstitions and to cart the child off to some strange den, certainly dirty, unhygienic and highly dangerous for small children who were prone to catch all kinds of infections! I was ashamed of my own pusillanimity, but my little boy kept screaming all the time. Thus, keeping it a secret from my parents, we took him to the *babka* anyway.

The healer turned out to be a stout woman in her mid-forties, who received us in her tiny apartment in a prefabricated apartment block, in one of the numerous vast areas of Moscow's '*novostroiki*', recently constructed on the site of outlying villages, but already dilapidated and slum-like in appearance. She asked us to wait in the small dark hall by the door, from where her humble quarters could be glimpsed. She took the baby into her room, where icons were hanging and an oil icon-lamp (*lampada*) was burning (which, at the time, although not entirely unusual, was still rather exotic to my eye). She put the baby on the table under the icons, unswaddled him, smeared his hernia with the sunflower oil that we had been instructed to bring with us, and muttered something almost inaudible, spells or prayers or a mixture of these, making quick movements with her fingers over the afflicted spot. The treatment took no more than five minutes and cost us five roubles. The woman asked us to visit her twice more for repeated treatment, but the third visit was not needed. In a couple of days, the hernia was gone, never to return.

This recollection from the Soviet period serves to illustrate the multiplicity of medical systems in Russia at that time, and the pragmatic attitude of users when they ran up against real problems, despite the dominant ideology that underlay therapeutic choices. Even back then, several health-seeking options were available. Simplifying for the sake of analysis, one can say that they fell into three broad categories that could be distinguished from one another both in terms of explanations and typologies of illness and in terms of the ideological (or cosmological) bases of treatment, as well as in terms of the sociology of practitioners and users. These categories are useful to consider in greater detail as they provided the genesis for the pluralistic field of healthcare that characterises today's Russia (described in closer detail in Lindquist 2002b).

Folk medicine

One is what later came to be labelled as 'folk medicine' (my own early encounter with its representative was, as we have seen above, quite gratifying). Even though folk magico-medical practices were officially (and even popularly, by some circles of users) sneered at and vilified as superstition, folk healing survived and was passed through generations, unobtrusively thriving in villages and in the working-class neighbourhoods of big cities. This folk tradition, borne by local healers, consisted of several elements.

There was a rich repertoire of folk remedies, utilising household means at hand, such as sunflower oil, honey, onion and mustard, as well as potions, brews and concoctions of herbs, roots and vegetables. These were ingested as drinks and laid on various parts of the body as compresses, embrocations and poultices. These folk remedies were widely used in families, irrespective of the social background, and the prescriptions, some of them quite elaborate, were the subject of a lively exchange between friends and relatives.

Folk medicine also used various types of para-ritual actions that were central to the repertoires of many folk healers. These rituals were idiosyncratic to individual healers, although they contained a number of common elements, notably manipulations with church candles and tapers (and other church paraphernalia), sprinkling with water which had been blessed, and various styles of reading prayers, spells and incantations. Prayers came from prayer books officially acknowledged by the Church, as well as from apocryphal sources that had survived from older times before prayer books had been standardised. There were also texts from folk poetry generated locally and handed down through relatives and neighbourhood healers. This highly expressive oral poetic heritage (described in Kharitonova 1995, among many others) had been collected by Russian ethnologists in pre-Soviet and Soviet times, and was available in specialised academic publications. These texts were also kept by individual healers as private collections, to be used in their own practices. Thus preserved, this body of texts was not forbidden in Soviet times, but it was nonetheless somewhat esoteric, limited in its distribution to specialised academic publications and private handwritten notebooks.

Whatever the parts of the ritual, they were optional and auxiliary to the main element of healing: the movements of the healer's hands over the body of the patient, and, specifically, over its afflicted part(s) – as was the case in my own encounter with the *babka* described above.

Bio-energy healing and studies of the paranormal

These movements over the body by hands or fingers, combined with prolonged touching, massage and bone-setting manipulations, are also central to the activities of the category that, for simplicity's sake, can be termed 'bio-field healers'.[4] Among this category of healer hand movements are stripped, partly or totally, of the ritual and textual paraphernalia characteristic of village wizards. Bio-field healing, and the people who practised it, *'ekstrasensy'*, proliferated unofficially in

Soviet times. Some biomedical practitioners discovered and developed these abilities in themselves and practised them along with other more conventional methods. For example, in the 1980s I knew a dentist who used these methods for anaesthesia and for treating abscesses and inflammations. There were many rumours about the famous Dzhuna, a Georgian healer who for many years kept Brezhnev alive, and about people like her, employed to treat the aging top Party leaders.

These phenomena of healing, which constitute a part of what is broadly labelled 'the unknown', have long fascinated the Russian popular and scientific imagination alike. In Soviet times, research into the paranormal was said to be performed in special laboratories under the aegis of the KGB, in cooperation and in competition with the CIA, as the folk tales still have it. There are written and oral accounts of people with paranormal abilities being connected to apparatuses, measured, and monitored through repeated experiments (see note 2). Today's healers still talk about these studies. An informant, for example, told me about a colleague of hers, who at some point worked closely with KGB researchers. As a part of the research programme, this man, she asserted, was asked to read papers in the locked safes in the US embassy, and to use his clairvoyance to draw maps of classified sites such as American military bases in Europe. Such cooperation, according to many healers, was far from innocent: once one agreed to cooperate, one was trapped. Such people, it is said, in the end died horrible deaths or disappeared.

Non-Russian medical traditions

Another category of alternative medical culture in Russia was represented by established nonbiomedical traditions, notably homeopathy, acupuncture and Ayur-Vedic and Tibetan medicine. Hypnotherapy and elements of psychoanalysis were taught and practised, but they were private, semi-underground, and known by a select few, mostly to circles of urban intelligentsia. Chiropractic and osteopathy overlapped with the traditional Russian folk art of bone-setting and massage (known in Russia as 'manual therapy' – *manuali'naia terapiia*) that was used by many village healers. Chinese and Indian medical techniques were introduced by members of ethnic communities, who came along with their compatriots – students, workers, and traders – to live in Russia during Soviet times.

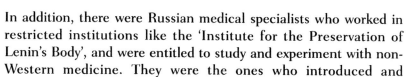

In addition, there were Russian medical specialists who worked in restricted institutions like the 'Institute for the Preservation of Lenin's Body', and were entitled to study and experiment with non-Western medicine. They were the ones who introduced and developed these arts.

In Soviet times these disciplines were practised privately, semi-secretly: they were not legally punishable, but neither were they widely advertised. ('Closed institutions of a well-known type' [*zakrytyie zavedeniia khorosho izvestnogo tipa*] still exist and stir popular imagination. They are still associated with the activity of magi and healers, and this fact is used in marketing to boost the image of the magus, as mentioned in Pachenkov 2001). The practitioners were mostly people with medical, technical and scientific college education, and they combined these methods with modern Western biomedicine. They adapted these methods to local conditions and worked on inventing machines and apparatuses based on related principles. Two of the most widely used of these machines are the AMSAD program for computer diagnostics and the Fol' apparatus. (The former is described in Chapter 5, and the latter in Samosiuk et al. 1994). A variety of these can be encountered in every large pharmacy in Moscow, where for a modest sum (100 roubles in 1999) a passer-by can receive a complete diagnosis of her health status.

Complementary medicine in post-perestroika Russia

These elements of nonbiomedical healthcare described above (folk medicine, bio-field healing with its para-scientific applications, and non-Western medical traditions) were thus in place even before perestroika. The greatest change that came with the demise of communism and the new freedoms was that all these practices took on clear visibility in the suddenly opening public arenas. Healers of all descriptions started to advertise in newspapers, and information about them, self-crafted or compiled by journalists, became available on radio and on TV. From being underground, and somewhat dubious from the ideological point of view, healing suddenly came out of the closet, as it were. Initially, in the early 1990s, it almost acquired the character of mass hysteria.

One of the best-known names, amongst others, was Kashpirovski. He was a psychologist, hypnotherapist and medical doctor who claimed to be able to heal all diseases in all people. He gave séances in huge stadiums in the largest cities of Russia, which were relayed by television to millions of enraptured observers. TV viewers could see on their screens people in the audience falling into trance, shaking and rocking and wringing their hands. As a part of the séance, Kashpirovski read out letters from grateful patients, reporting miraculous recoveries from incurable diseases. In addition, people brought with them bottles of water that the healer 'charged with his energy', to be used as a remedy from whatever diseases one suffered from. TV viewers were instructed to put vessels with water in front of their television screens, so that they could be 'charged' during the broadcast. While watching, they were instructed to concentrate on their particular diseases, or on those of their loved ones, even if the afflicted persons themselves were not physically present in front of the TV. The healing energy of Kashpirovski was supposed to be transmitted, not only via the physical medium of water, but also through the bodies and the intentions of family members concerned about their loved ones.

Kashpirovski's popularity did not last long, however. He was accused of involvement in financial and sexual scandals, was sued, and eventually forced to leave the country. As to his healing potential, more and more people accused him, not of being ineffective, but of aggravating the conditions of those exposed to his treatment. Rumours started that ambulance services were overly full after his mass séances: people got acute attacks of the conditions they had suffered from chronically or latently. The healing power of a charismatic person, concentrated, multiplied, and amplified through modern mass media, finally changed the sign and became the power of evil, not so much eliminating as aggravating diseases, not healing but harming. Perhaps Russians in fact had grown tired of mega-scale charismatic leaders, who promised to solve all problems with one piercing glance at a faceless crowd, holding an unquestioning belief. Kashpirovski's charisma, which had initially seemed overwhelming, proved to be insufficient, and eventually he had to quit.

Several other healers who ventured to perform on a mass scale also quickly left the stage. Some reappeared after many years as private persons, catering not for a mass of people, but rather for smaller groups of followers, connected to their leaders through more personal relationships. One of these people was Chumak, who had been a big-time radio and TV-healer, and who reappeared ten years later in a small newspaper advertisement promoting his mail-order business. Now he was selling face and body creams charged with his energy, promising that these would bestow on their users the divine energy of the Cosmos, mediated by the healer. These would give their users not only health and well-being but also prolonged youth and beauty. Thus, in one decade his project metamorphosed from grand-scale ideas for the wholesale salvation of Russia through the healing power of one individual, to a commercial mail-order beauty business.

In the meantime, many specialists of the kinds mentioned in the previous section also appeared more publicly, attempting to make a living from their healing arts. In Soviet times, folk healers and other practitioners had jobs paid by the State and practised healing on the side. Many of these jobs now had ceased to exist or could not provide incomes sufficient for survival. Many men, and especially women, started to advertise all kinds of magical and healing services. These advertisements reflect the strategies that practitioners employ to forge legitimacy and to define the circles of their potential clients. Elsewhere I have termed these references to the domains of meaning accepted by people of different social circles 'strategies of legitimation' (Lindquist 2001b; see also MacCormack 1981, 1986). They are essential for the practitioners' personal charisma, and are briefly discussed below.

Reference to the scientific establishment

As has been already mentioned, there is a category of healers who have official licences, and who work in clinics. They depend on the biomedical health care system for the renewal of their licences, as well as for other everyday interactions. In addition, such people refer to conventional science and biomedicine in order to forge meaning and legitimacy. It is clearly seen in the newspaper advertisements, also described by Pachenkov for St Petersburg. Thus, the text of one of them states[5]:

> Grigorii Grabovoi graduated from the Faculty of Applied Mathematics and Mechanics, Tashkent University, and obtained a medical degree in Moscow, specialising in general therapy. He discovered a region of creation [the ad does not disclose what that is], the discovery of which is patented. Grigorii Petrovich is a member of the International Information Academy, the New York Academy of Sciences, the Russian Academy of Medico-Technical

Sciences. He is an honorary member of the Russian Academy of Cosmonautics, a Doctor of Technical Sciences, a Doctor of Philosophy, a member of the Professional League of Psychotherapists [This list of distinctions continues for half a page, containing dozens of other titles and degrees from Russian and foreign associations, leagues, and academies.]

This advertisement concludes with 'Moscow Health Care Committee Licence No.'

Such references to scientific degrees are interspersed with parascientific terminology. Sometimes, the language of the scientifically conceived paranormal prevails. Healers qualify themselves as 'Progressor' or 'Magister of Cosmo-energetics', and offer 'Purification and treatment with the help of Divine Cosmic Energy, irrespective of nationality and faith. Without the use of medicines, prayers, spells, incantations, or hypnosis.' Others may include the mention of international distinctions: 'Parapsychologist, bioenergotherapist, clairvoyant, magus, international hypnologist'. Or, a practitioner can qualify himself as a 'folk healer, natural holy planetary healer, the official member of the international register [the type of the register is not mentioned], bioenergotherapist, eniooperator, clairvoyant, physiotherapist, cytologist, candidate of biological sciences' (quoted by Pachenkov 2001 from *Zerkalo Peterburga*, No. 1, February 1997).

Reference to the 'Russian roots'

Another strategy adopted by healers and magi is to advertise themselves as 'folk' healers' (*narodnyi tselitel'*) and as heirs to the village wizards. Legitimacy here is traditional, the thread of wisdom coming from the mystical *narod* or people. In advertisements, this fact can be stated concisely, in the title introducing the person, e.g. 'Aksinia – hereditary healer'. Or, the advertisement text, which might well go on at length, may present the healer's genealogy in a more evocative way:

> For centuries the Razviazkin lineage has been famous for its healers. This hereditary line of healers was renowned far and wide, many people having trodden the path to their house. When Sergei was born on the holy day of the Baptism of Christ, in raging cold, everybody realised: he was not only continuing the lineage, he was also an heir to secret knowledge. His destiny, like that of his grandfather, great grandfather, and all his ancestors, was to heal people, to save them from their troubles and misfortunes.

In the background of the photograph there is a huge crucifix, with another massive cross on the healer's chest. He holds a crystal ball and a magic lantern in his hands.

Here we see how many healers (and magi), like this one, refer to God, faith and religion, either in very direct terms, or, more subtly, through using Russian Orthodox Church paraphernalia, in conjunction with legitimation through the 'folk tradition', and in order to augment the reference to the 'roots'. For example, a very concise advertisement introduces 'a folk healer', who promises to 'cure all diseases in one séance'. Instead of lists of degrees and distinctions, references to scientific publications and licence numbers, there is one single phrase: 'Faith in God will heal you!' Advertisements feature an establishment referred to as 'the Center of Russian Orthodox Religious Healing'; a healer who heals through 'Russian Orthodox prayers from the Church prayer books', and so forth. This kind of blend, however, is quite contentious, in view of the already mentioned deep resentment that the Church has against all kinds of healing and magic (Lindquist 2000a).

Reference to alterity

Finally, a large group of magi and healers trace their charismatic provenance to foreign magical practices. One advertisement introduces 'The parlour [*salon*] of Supreme Magic presided by Selene Vamp, the heir of Ancient Babylonian teachings to the seventh generation, Magister of Black Magic and Voodoo, Knight of the Order of the 10th Legion, of the Three Winds.' There is a hereditary Scythian priestess and there is a Magister of Indian and Tibetan Medicine. There is 'Tamara Asgard – the only one in Russia who masters the secret techniques of ancient Scandinavian runic symbols.' Another centre offers 'all kinds of sorcery, from primitive Voodoo and Wicca to Supreme Magic'. 'Reiki – for those who seek spiritual power, a Japanese tradition to extract the vital force, to become one with it, and to transmit it through your hands'; 'The Supreme Voodoo priest Seraphim Kassandré, blessed by the Great Voodoo Priest Babalua Vonban Kanbobo'. (For more on Voodoo magic in Moscow, see Lindquist 2001d). There is a 'Higher Priest of Pagan cults, shaman-parapsychologist of international class, adept of the Black Moon Mystery'; there are Celtic and Egyptian priestesses; and many more besides. In Moscow there is at least one very popular

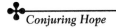

and successful 'neo-shaman', a student of Michael Harner, who helps her clients to journey to the underworld and to find their 'Power Animals' (see Lindquist 2002a). Harnerian drum journeys undertaken by the practising healers themselves, as part of their formal training at 'courses', are described in Kharitonova 1999.

From this background of magic and healing as an integral constituent of the urban landscape, I shall turn to specific establishments, and to individual practitioners who work within them (or outside of them, as the case may be, all on their own in the Moscow 'jungle'). In the remainder of this chapter, I shall offer a closer look at the social organisation of a particular business unit offering magic and healing services in market conditions: a Centre, or Salon, of Magic. I shall look at some practitioners working in the field, homing in on one of them in particular; and at an instance of interaction between a 'specialist' and a client. That will give an initial idea of how the practitioners construct themselves as icons of power, intersubjectively, through their dealings with clients and with their fellow practitioners. This will also develop the argument set out at the beginning of this chapter, namely that magic services represent a segment of the market that gives employment to enterprising individuals, gifted in a certain way. This sector of the newly emerged market economy offers goods and services that are in high demand, but it also fosters this very demand through mechanisms that combine rational strategies of economic agents with emotional impulses and manipulations: market and magic are bedfellows as close (albeit maybe as uneasy) as rationality and emotions.

A site of the magic industry: the 'Centaur' centre

'Centaur' (a pseudonym), a centre, or a clinic, of magic and healing, is one of a vast array of enterprises that sell their services in supposedly market conditions: the purchasers pay for the work (and products) that the sellers provide. Tatiana is employed in this centre: she goes there every day, five days a week (and sometimes more), to receive clients, and draws her monthly salary, paid by the owner of the centre. In this respect, she differs from most other specialists portrayed in this book, i.e. individual entrepreneurs who have to survive in the new 'jungle' entirely on their own.

Tatiana's story

Tatiana has a reputation for healing diseases of the spine and bones, being able to straighten crooked spines or protruding shoulder blades, remove lameness, stretch one leg that is shorter than the other, increase the length of the body by up to ten centimetres as well as remove hunches in the back. Thus, Tatiana's magical powers are concentrated on the area of matter, on the physical body, along with the mind and psyche. Accordingly, in the advertisements she figures primarily as a healer rather than a magus.

Tatiana came from a working-class family, and started her professional life as a draughtswoman in a technical designer's office (*konstruktorskoie biuro*), designing tractors and other agricultural machinery, a secure, comfortable job. At the end of the 1980s, however, the tractor-building industry collapsed, as did many other industries, burying under the rubble many research and development establishments, institutes and offices like Tatiana's.

At that time, when the spectre of starvation seemed for many to lurk on the horizon, she found herself unemployed, with a teenage son and without her husband who had just left her for another woman. Like many healers, Tatiana had 'magic hands': she liked to soothe and console, and her colleagues in the design bureau would usually ask her to cure their headaches and other small ailments. She used all her savings to take one of the many courses on massage and bone-setting that started to proliferate in Moscow at that time, and she turned out to be quite good at it.

After graduating from her courses with the certificate of a licensed masseur, she found work in a district polyclinic, taking blood samples and giving injections. On her home visits, in addition to injections and massage, she started to practice hand healing, which her patients greatly appreciated. A patient advised her to try her luck at an institute for Folk and Alternative Medicine, one of the first establishments of the kind in Moscow. Presided over by a professor of psychology with a keen eye for business, this Institute admitted 'folk healers' and people with 'paranormal abilities' who had already gained some repute, educated them in biomedicine, and gave them a certificate in 'folk healing'.

The entrance test consisted of, among other things, diagnosing a patient with the help of her 'X-ray vision'. Tatiana looked at the patient, at his complexion, his posture, felt his bio-field with her hands, and diagnosed liver cirrhosis, which turned out to be correct. When she graduated a year later, she was a certified 'folk healer' and, as such, she finally got employed in 'Centaur'.

'Centaur'

The 'Centaur' centre is five minutes' walk from a subway station, occupying spacious premises on the first floor of a grey brick building. The sign, conspicuous from all directions, presents the place as a *'salon magii'*, in contrast to the alternative widespread designation of similar centres, dealing mainly with rehabilitation and the treatment of physical diseases – *lechebno-ozdorovitel'nyi tsentr* or *klinika*. Such clinics draw their legitimacy from self-consciously constructed associations with the health-care system, and bring to mind the serious business of disease treatment. The label *'salon'*, on the other hand, suggests the more luxurious side of life; not treating diseases but rather beautifying the outward appearance. *'Salon'* means 'parlour', and in its Russian usage refers to hairdressers, skin care or beauty parlours, or to more expensive tailoring shops (as in the *'salon modnoi odezhdy'*, clothing and sewing ateliers where women with better financial means in Soviet times could order personally designed and tailored clothes).

Indeed, the Centaur magic parlour looks more like a business office than a clinic. One enters a corridor that serves as a waiting room, equipped with comfortable sofas and armchairs. The first person one encounters at the entrance is the guard, an athletic-looking figure stationed in front of a TV monitor that shows the flight of stairs leading to the entrance.[6] At the end of the corridor there is the room for the secretaries, three young beauties, complete with long legs, vanishingly small skirts, expensive make-up, and equipped with state-of-the-art headphone sets with tiny microphones, to answer the telephone calls on three lines.

Some clients who ring Centaur wish to see only the magi they have already been working with. Many clients, however, are trying out the establishment for the first time, and during this initial call they will only vaguely indicate the nature of their problems. In this case it is the job of the secretaries to refer the prospective clients to the 'specialists', the staff magi. The number of clients has a direct bearing on the amount of money earned by the magi, and so the secretaries have a certain power over the centre's specialists. On the other hand, as Tatiana intimated, the secretaries are only pawns of the boss, the young businessman who is the director of the centre, and to whom all the staff are directly subordinate.

A glass show-case exhibiting samples of talismans for sale is conspicuous in the waiting-room: semi-precious stones such as turquoise, tiger eye, marble and malachite, as well as stitched leather bags with strings or strips of leather. Clients in the hall waiting to be shown in to the magi have a chance to take a good look at the amulets, whose price in 1999 varied from 700 to 2,000 roubles. The price list for the basic services provided is displayed near the cashier's desk: the first, diagnostic consultation costs 500 roubles, whereas the price of treatments is not specified, but varies according to the seriousness of the problem and the difficulty of the work to be completed. (These prices were for 1999 when the fieldwork was done. For comparison, an average salary at the time was 1,500 roubles, a pension or the minimum wage 800 roubles, and the rate of the rouble to the dollar 29 : 1.)

In a corner of the secretarys' room there is a computer, and clients are routinely sent by magi to undergo a computer diagnostic. For an additional 200 roubles (in addition to the standard initial consultation fee) they receive a coloured picture of their spine and vertebrae, where the colours correspond to the seriousness of the affliction of their inner organs and viscera. Magi require that their clients take this picture irrespective of the nature of their complaint, in case any further work needs to be done; it is the equivalent of a regular medical test run in a biomedical clinic. Even if a client complains, say, of love or family problems, which seemingly have nothing to do with her health, the computer diagnostic is said to show purely physical disturbances at an early stage, which will make it easier for the magus to then work holistically, and alleviate the problems in their totality. This approach is not unfamiliar to Russian patients, as sending people for blood tests, ultrasound scans and X-rays, irrespective of the nature of their complaints, has always been a widespread practice in biomedical clinics. Tatiana (who, of course, asked her patients to have the same tests done) confided in me, however, that, in her opinion, this was totally unnecessary, just one of the many ways devised by the bosses of the centre (*'nachal'stvo'*) to squeeze money out of people.

The pragmatics of magic on the micro levels of survival

As I discuss in detail elsewhere, some magi see themselves as moral leaders and the spiritual teachers called on to bring about the evolution of the world, or at least of Russia (Lindquist, 2000b, and Chapter 4, this volume.) The clients, however, are mostly not interested in questions of an abstractly spiritual nature. Alongside all their other lofty targets, magi are above all professionals who have to survive on their craft. Therefore, they offer help where it is sought, that is, on the micro level of everyday survival, equally tough for Russians from all walks of life. The minute practicality of the problems solved magically stands out strikingly in the case of one particular magus, who is highly successful, advertised lavishly in the media, and regularly gives courses and draws a full house in the big movie theatres. Raisa Ryk (this is her real name, often seen on the big billboards and in the headlines of newspapers) has a page in every issue of the newspaper *Tainaia vlast*, where she addresses her followers in what appears to be a particularly unabashed extolling of her magical crafts and powers, reminiscent of the Western television evangelist miracle-makers (see. e.g. Coleman 2000). Besides the usual promises of 'the codes of love and luck', Raisa Ryk purports to supply her students with specialised magical skills highly conducive to everyday survival. Large parts of the accounts she provides as advertisement are narratives of the feats achieved by the people empowered by her magical force, which became theirs through personal contact, by telephone, or through the lectures or courses that she regularly gives:

> An eleven-year-old girl who attended my courses together with her mother once found herself in a subway car where seven people were about to start a violent row. Not only did she stop the fighters in five minutes, but she also made them shake hands and leave the subway-car through different doors and disappear in different directions. A 12-year-old boy succeeded in immediately bringing a policeman into the carriage of a late night suburban train when a drunken hooligan started to harass the passengers.

There was a woman who had lent 2,000 dollars to an acquaintance, and had not been able to get it back for two years. After a course with me, she took my book [a book written by Raisa], put it under her pillow and kept saying throughout the night: 'Raisa, help me! Let my neighbour give me back the 2,000 dollars she has borrowed!' The next day the neighbour turned up with the money.

A woman who had gone through my courses was once walking alone, and suddenly she felt a chill on her back. When she turned around she saw a man with a knife running after her. In her thoughts, she instantly put up a protective barrier, and the man tripped and fell, cursed, and turned back.

Among other services, Raisa Ryk offers to 'see which bank it is safe to put your money into, [and to] look over (*prosmotret'*) your business partner [whether he is a reliable person and is not going to rob you of your money], an investment, or a business trip.' She can also tell you how (if indeed at all) a missing person met his death, if it was violent and painful, and where you can find the body. 'You draw up a mental image of the person, and check his neck and his lungs. If you feel that there is a rope on his neck or his lungs are heavy, it means that he was strangled or hanged'.

Raisa Ryk encourages her students and clients to use her photograph, reprinted in every issue of the newspaper, to infuse with her energy all their physical entourage and material possessions – it may be their wallets, the water that they drink and that they use at their vegetable gardens, the seeds they sow, their papers when they travel abroad, and the school report books of their children. I have seen Raisa Ryk's portrait amongst other places in a car owned by Misha, a Moscow acquaintance and one of my main informants, who will appear later on these pages. The car was so old and battered that the mere fact it was moving at all seemed magical: an occurrence where 'natural laws' are suspended and unknown forces (*nepozannnoie*) come into play. When Misha climbed into his car, he was never sure whether it would start again. The fact that it did was always a minor miracle. You cannot expect a miracle to happen, but you can always hope (here, it is pertinent to recall that hope is an ungrounded faith in a good outcome, according to Hart 1988). Raisa Ryk's portrait on the radiator of Misha's car can be compared with small images of patron saints and miracle-making icons of Our Lady that you can see in many vehicles in Russian as well as Latin American and Mediterranean cities: the last resort, someone who helps when all the rest fails; an icon of power and a token of hope.

45

It has been argued that the practices of magic and sorcery persist in societies where the uncertainty of existence is exceedingly high (Whyte 1998). In post-Communist Russia, uncertainty permeates everyday life all the way down to its micro levels. In this life, nothing can be taken for granted, and trivial everyday occurrences become daring adventures with miraculous outcomes. These miracles are often accounted for by the involvement of magical elements (or, for pious people, are explained by the benevolence of God).

In the natural course of events, neither banks nor neighbours return loans; policemen do not appear after the first call in a late-night suburban train; and street violence does not stop by the attackers changing their minds or by their suddenly tripping up and turning back. There is a multitude of situations, of varying import for the lives of those involved, with varying degrees of humiliation ensuing, and with various implications for survival; but all of them are equally out of the actors' control by any 'rational' social means, physical or legal. Magic is a social means that makes uncertainty bearable and hope possible.

The advertisements of Raisa Ryk quote satisfied users who report a number of such minor miracles on the micro level of everyday practice. 'The clock, coffee grinding machine, TV and the car-wipers suddenly started working after Raisa's course'; 'Many thanks – I have no more problems with the traffic police'; 'You helped me to get back the things that had been stolen'; 'My children made it up with each other and stopped drinking'; 'I found the body of my friend exactly where you told me'; and even 'I exterminated cockroaches in my apartment with the help of your picture'. Here, the power with which the magus is imbued can take both a positive and a negative charge, depending on the task; it can boost and multiply (money or harvest), as well as weaken and destroy (cockroaches, kidney stones or violent attackers).

Similarly, the eulogy-advertisements in the home newspaper of 'Centaur' recount success stories of miraculous cures.

An amusing little old man is dancing wildly in the waiting room, cheerfully kicking the air with his scrawny little legs [*zabavnyi starichok otpliasyvaiet v priemnoi, veselo vskidyvaia sukhonkie nozhki*]. Liudmila, on the way to her office, tries to pass by without drawing attention to herself. 'Don't you remember me?' asks the old man merrily. 'I came to you on crutches the first time'. Indeed she does not remember him: so many people come to seek her help. What you tend to remember [as a magus] is difficult cases, cases that look hopeless, something that took hard work [healing a crippled old man so that he can dance wildly was such an easy job that it did not even register in the magus's memory].

When Vasilii first came to Zinaida [the magus], his hands were trembling, his eyes bloodshot, his face gaunt and unshaven. His business had collapsed, he was drinking heavily, and his wife had just taken their child and moved out to her mother's apartment. Now Vasilii is a strong and handsome man with a fresh complexion, exuding masculinity [*muzhestvennost'*] and self-confidence. His newly revived business has several branches, some of them abroad, and his wife, back with him, is expecting another baby. Vasilii is sitting in the waiting room with his bodyguards: success makes you vulnerable. But, according to him, bodyguards are an extra, just in case: it is from Zinaida that he gets the real protection. He never parts with the stone she once gave him. This time he came to Zinaida in order to get help in the up-coming election campaign: he will run as a candidate to the Duma from his native province. He knows that with Zinaida behind him, he cannot fail. (*Tainaia sila* No. 4 1999).

The little scarf of bad luck

In real life, the stories of treatment may sound somewhat different, especially as seen from the client's perspective. Misha, the owner of the miraculously working car mentioned above, happened at some point to have been a client of Zinaida, a magus working at Centaur and enjoying an awesome reputation. He came to Zinaida with the last 700 roubles he had earned by driving people around. He had heard about her from a friend and called for an appointment. Before being shown in, he had to leave 500 roubles with the cashier. He thought Zinaida was an impressive woman, with authority and knowledge. But when he tried to tell his story, she sternly interrupted him, saying that this was unnecessary, because she saw already very clearly what was the matter with Misha. The problem, according to her, was 'the little scarf of bad luck' [*sharfik nevezeniia*] wound around his neck. The virtual scarf, invisible to all except Zinaida, who had magic eyesight, acted as a strangling rope, blocking the channels between the divine energy of the cosmos and Misha's astral and physical body. She also noticed that he had no protection, and that his energy field had a breach through which the energy was constantly leaking. She said that she had to restore the protection, and to this effect, as an initial measure, she ordered that Misha buy a stone, a tiger's eye. The stone cost 300 roubles, payable to the cashier. He said that he had only 200 left, and Zinaida conceded that she could give him a discount, selling him one of her own private stones, charged with her energy. He told me that he was disappointed by the quick and noncommittal manner in which she reached into the drawer of her desk and produced a stone, without even looking at it. Without further ceremony, she handed the stone to Misha, instructing him always to keep it next to his body, and never show it to anyone, much less to let anyone touch it (lest people's evil eyes and envious intentions destroy its magic protective qualities). She said that the stone was the first, crucial, but by no means sufficient, step towards bettering his situation, and that she had to work on Misha over several séances.

Misha did not have the money for more séances, nor did he feel much desire to go back to Zinaida, put off by her bossy and nonchalant manner. But now he physically felt the wretched little scarf tied around his neck. He perceived it so vividly that he was almost suffocated, and he was convinced that no good could happen to him with this scarf around his neck. So, he asked the magus to remove the scarf before he left. Zinaida told him dryly that removing the scarf would require a session, which would take another appointment at a totally different rate; what was going on now was only a diagnostic consultation. She added that his protection field was so weak (even with the stone on) that the scarf would come back in no time. Misha insisted that he did not care if the scarf came back later, he wanted it to be taken away there and then, and he could not pay any more. The magus said that the time was up (*priem okonchen*), and that if he wanted the job done he should come back soon, no more than a couple of days later. She looked him right in the eyes with what he experienced as a vague menace, and he obediently walked out of her room. After that 'diagnostic consultation', he constantly felt the tight grip of the scarf around his neck. The presence of the stone, however, reassured him to a degree; and Zinaida told him on his way out that he was sufficiently protected by the stone, so nothing really terrible would happen to him.

This was Misha's first and last visit to Zinaida. He became trapped in a situation where he had a chronic lack of money, living from day to day with hardly enough to pay his second-hand rent for an apartment that he shared with three other men, or to buy the gasoline for his car, his only source of income. Misha's situation changed for the better only after he met Katerina, and became her devoted friend and follower – but this is another story, to be told later.

Microeconomics of Centaur

What is relevant to my discussion here, and crucial for the economy of Centaur, is the ease with which magus Zinaida made her client part with all his money, beyond the amount officially needed for the visit. Physically strangled by the virtual little scarf of bad luck, Misha was bound to come back as many times as she deemed necessary. He would probably have done it if he had had the money: he was never in any doubt about her authority as a magus, or about her magical power. What repelled him was the lack of dedicated, personalised human attention, the absence of a human bond that he later found with Katerina. This impression was augmented by the shortness of the time Zinaida devoted to him. As my informant Tatiana told me, Zinaida was highly regarded in the centre precisely because of her high processing capacity: the amount of clients going through her during the day was maybe five times higher than that for Tatiana herself. Of course, this was Tatiana's perspective, naturally tainted by exasperation and – as even magi are only human – maybe a fraction of envy. In Zinaida's rendering the whole story would certainly be totally different. Unfortunately, I was not lucky enough to have Zinaida among my informants.

On a different note, the reasons for Zinaida's clear advantage over Tatiana in terms of her money-producing capacity can be understood with regard to Tatiana's speciality, the treatment of bone diseases, a process that is always based on long and careful massages. However, in spite of the diverging nature of their treatments, and of the difference in terms of time and effort required, the price charged for the treatment was the same, 800 roubles, the price set by the centre based on the market price of similar services from other establishments currently available in Moscow at that time. Thus, Zinaida's productivity was five times as high as Tatiana's, and so was her worth for the centre. Tatiana was bitter about the centre and about her colleagues, whom she called greedy charlatans who sold their magical talents for money. Zinaida, and magi like her, according to Tatiana, were openly favoured by the centre. Their ability, quoting Tatiana, to 'impose unnecessary rubbish on people' ('*vsuchat' liudiam vsiakuiu drian*''), such as the stone sold to Misha, obviously only enhanced their reputations, and multiplied the favours poured on them by the director. Those favours included more days off; the amount of advertisement space in the newspaper and the frequency of the ads' appearance; larger rooms, new equipment such as lamps, chairs and shelves; and many other more subtle but perceptible things.

But the most important discrimination strategy was the allocation of patients. Although this was formally done by the secretaries, everybody knew that the informal decisions were made by the director himself. In the difficult times following the financial crisis of 1998 the scarce and precious clients were channelled to Zinaida instead of Tatiana, provided that they did not have the special problems that were Tatiana's hallmark. Clients with love problems, for example, who needed only a simple ritual for augmenting attractiveness, a couple of spells and a stone, were always sent to Tatiana's colleagues and rivals. As a result, her fellow Centaur magi were earning many times more than Tatiana, even though they, according to Tatiana, retained only a third of what the clients paid (the rest went to the 'blood-sucking director', a successful businessman apparently juggling with many balls). In addition, their small illegalities, like selling a stone without the knowledge of the cashier, were tacitly tolerated.

At the time of my fieldwork the number of such centres had declined markedly following the crisis of August 1998, as only the most successful people could afford to run centres that, after all, did not bring in much income. The director of Centaur was, according to Tatiana, a real exploiter. She claimed that the working rooms were all supplied with watch holes (*glazok*) through which the director and his henchmen could make random checks on the magi, to make sure that they did not make private appointments, exchange telephone numbers, sell amulets, overrun the time of the treatment, receive additional money from the clients, etc. Of course, none of this could be completely controlled, as Russian people are experts in cheating their employers. This is a useful survival skill that they have retained from Soviet times, when the only employer was the State (see Birdsall 2000). However, despite all her grievances, Tatiana had at the time no intention of leaving the centre and starting to work on her own.

In later chapters, I shall describe other healers, who operate on the market not as dependent employees, like Tatiana, but as free entrepreneurs: either licensed and registered, in the framework of officially recognised institutions, or unregistered and untied to any institutions, totally on their own. But before doing so, I shall look at the terms of affliction and methods of treatment in terms of semiotic processes in which they are involved. In the next chapter, I shall explore how words, objects and ritual actions that constitute healing and magic might do their work of intersubjective transformations of clients' embodied consciousness.

Notes

1. The term 'nontraditional' (*netradistionnyi*), used in official Russian parlance as applied to the methods of treatment outside conventional biomedicine, appears confusing. It denotes a broad spectrum of approaches to health care, from acupuncture and herbal medicine to bone-setting and metaphysical and faith healing, sometimes referred to as 'bio-sensorics'. 'Tradition' implied in this usage of the term 'nontraditional' refers here not to folk traditions of healing, as could be expected, but, instead, to 'new' or 'modern' ways of biomedicine that by the end of the twentieth century were supposed to become 'traditional' for a generic inhabitant of Russia. Another, synonymic term, used to denote the same area of health care, is 'complementary medicine'. The implication of this term is that the methods concerned are used as a complement to biomedical practices, which is quite legitimate in Russia, and which is in fact often the case both in regular (especially private) biomedical clinics and in people's everyday practices.

2. There is much experimental and theoretical research into this and other kinds of 'paranormal' phenomena in Russia. One of its foremost representatives is Dr Valentina Kharitonova, ethnologist and folklorist from the Moscow Institute of Anthropology and Ethnology. She has studied magic and healing in urban and rural Russia, and in non-Russian parts of the Russian Federation both east and west of the capitals (in Ukraine and in Siberia) for the last twenty-five years. Her publications, both popular and academic, are extensive. Dr Kharitonova's work is based on similar ideational premises as that of the people she studies. These ideas, moreover, are shared by many representatives of natural sciences, such as biophysics, neurophysiology, quantum physics and biomedicine. Dr Kharitonova is engaged in an active research programme together with these disciplines, using technology to distinguish 'people with a real gift' from 'charlatans and those who are sincerely mistaken about their abilities'. The main thesis of Dr Kharitonova is that what she terms 'magico-medical practices' share a common ground. People with 'abilities', entering the Altered States of Consciousness, are able, through their 'psychic energy' or will, both to receive information from the 'field' (also called thin-matter plane [*tonkomaterial'nyi plan*]) and to alter this information, thus changing the reality. This line of thought is well known in the West, e.g. in the studies of 'shamanism'. The ethnography of folk magic practices, as a part of folklore

studies, is too abundant in Russia to review it here (detailed review of this literature is given in Ryan 1999). In their contemporary aspect, these practices have received attention from local and foreign students of revived indigenous shamanisms, which often coexist and overlap with the practices I describe in this book. Recent Russian-language literature on this subject is collected in several volumes edited by V. Kharitonova and D. Funk under the title 'Ethnological Studies of Shamanism and Other Traditional Beliefs and Practices', and in V. Kharitonova's 'The Art of Spells and Incantations of the Ancient Slavs', both published by the Moscow Institute of Ethnology and Anthropology throughout the 1990s. The best-known articles on shamanism in post-Soviet Siberia are Humphrey (2002), Vitebski (1995) and Balzer (1993).

3. In Pachenkov's analysis, magis' claim to solve these problems is a part of their marketing strategy, when they compete with other, nonmagical or 'rational' specialists such as business consultants, medical doctors and psychologists. Just like them, magi promise to solve people's most ordinary, everyday predicaments, although with nonordinary means. The way magi present themselves as approachable, recognisable and human is, according to Pachenkov, another part of this marketing strategy.

4. Kharitonova distinguishes between *supersensitive* abilities, responsible for perception by the 'senses not known to science'; and *extrasensorial* abilities, that enable people to affect the environment and other people by means of 'unusual' powers (*Avtoreferat dissertatsii*, published by the Moscow Institute of Ethnology and Anthropology, p. 30). The popular notion '*ekstrasens*' subsumes both modes of action.

5. All the texts of advertisements used in this chapter are taken from the newspapers *Orakul* and *Tainaia vlast* of 1999. All of them run continuously from one issue to another of these both newspapers for the whole year (some of these names were still seen in the years 2000 and 2001).

6. Such door guards are often part of the entourage of solid business offices. Their obvious function is to ward off robberies and violent attacks that are still among the principle means of settling business disagreements. This is a clear indication of the fact, hinted at by several of my informants, that such centres are merely the tips of business icebergs, and that they may serve as façades for more expansive and more shady businesses. One informant led me to believe that the centre she worked in was one of many convenient places for money laundering. However, in magic parlours these guards have the additional function of keeping away frustrated clients who come to demand their money back when the promised results of their investments into magic are not forthcoming.

Chapter 2
Magic as Semiotic Changes: Ontologies, Rituals and Terms of Affliction

So far, I have set the stage for magic as a profession, and as a service on the market. In this chapter, I shall consider interaction between the magus and the client as semiosis, manipulated by the magus in order to change the client's orientational dynamics – to alter the client's self. This process may start even before treatment proper is initiated, on the occasion of the first conversation between the magus and the client, when the diagnosis is made. I shall suggest that the terms of affliction, used to name the patient's problems, may have a potential to trigger transformation of the self already from the moment that they are uttered. The tools used in treatment – simple ritual and gestural performances – work in the same way as the terms used to define afflictions, namely iconically and indexically. They reshape emotions and attitudes – alter the experience of the self – leading to new bodily sensations and changed orientational engagements with the world.

It is an evening after a long working day for Inna, a professional Moscow magus. She receives her clients in a shabby two-room flat in a grey-brown brick apartment block. Inna, her friend Marina and myself are sitting in the kitchen, where the kettle is boiling on the stove, to brew the ubiquitous pot of black tea. Marina makes her living as an accountant in a small private company, but has a good working knowledge of *magia* and extra-sensorics, acquired from many years of studies from books and courses. She is also interested in psychology, and at present she is attending evening courses on the subject. Marina is a sturdy woman, accustomed to hard work, with a cheerful attitude and spiky good humour. But this evening she looks tired and dispirited, her face is drawn, her complexion greyish, her voice coarse. She tells us that she has had difficulties sleeping, that she catches colds all the time and can never get rid of one before the next one comes. She is haunted by short spells of bad luck, nothing terrible, but irritating and exhausting. She has made a couple of serious mistakes at work, and it is no wonder that her boss is angry with her. Besides this, her husband, a fairly successful businessman and usually a decent man, keeps coming home late, smelling strange, and snapping back at her when she asks where he has been. 'Please, check me up,' she asks Inna. 'I think it is *sglaz*, but I am not sure.'

Inna lifts her eyes from the tea mug and stares at Marina for a long while with a dark, concentrated gaze, as if transfixed.

'Yes, it is *sglaz*, and a rather well-advanced one,' she says at last. 'I see a young woman, dark-haired, next to Boria [Marina's husband]. She has been wishing you ill for quite some time, and it was only your strong protection that prevented it from developing into *porcha*.'

'Yes, he got a new secretary three months ago. I met her at that party ... Oh, I should have known! She was all sweetness, telling me how nice I looked in that red dress ... And the next week I broke my tooth, and then I hit my car, that's how it all started ...'

'So,' Inna concludes, 'it seems as if this young lady decided to arrange her life. At your expense. She will not succeed, don't worry. But before dealing with her, we must first work with you. We must take away the dirt she has been pumping there [into Marina's bio-field]. And we shall strengthen your protection.'

This episode captures the crucial part in the interaction between the magus and the client: the instance of diagnosing, when the client's condition receives a name. The afflicted person presents the problem; the magus responds by reformulating the client's predicament in the language of the typology of afflictions.

In healing practices, the human body is understood as being surrounded by some kind of 'bio-energy field' (*biopole*), organised by 'energo-information structures' (*energo-informatsionnyie struktury*) that work as programming mechanisms, and that are connected with the higher source of power through channels. These structures govern the functioning of internal organs, thus determining physical health. They also underlie the person's mental and emotional dispositions, shaping all the spheres of her life, her patterns of sociality, and the lives and fates of those close to her. These structures are in some way affected, not only by one's own deeds in this life (as is the case with the Buddhist notion of *karma*), but also by those of one's close ancestors. 'Bio-field' or *biopole* is now firmly part of the language, as well as 'energies', sometimes rendered as *energetika*. So are *negativy* (pl.; sing. *negativ*), the disturbances of the bio-field that are manifested by troubles in health and social life.

Sglaz, an effect of the evil eye, is a term well-known by scholars of Russian folk magic (Ivanits 1989; Ryan 1999). Belief in the evil eye is found in many parts of the world (for an overview, see Bowie 2000: 235–40). In pre-revolutionary Russia it was believed that any person who was recognised as a witch or wizard could cast an evil eye, as well as anyone with 'black, protruding, crossed or in some way distinctive eyes or otherwise peculiar appearance; [as well as] foreigners and priests' (Ryan 1999: 33). But evil eye could also be cast inadvertently: by 'injudicious praising', for example of one's baby or one's other precious possessions, such as health, clothes or general good luck (such as in the example above when the husband's secretary praised Marina's looks). One can even attract 'evil eye' upon oneself, for example by reckless boasting, which is considered as tempting fate. In common parlance, positive utterances regarding one's own life are habitually followed by saying *t'fu-t'fu – ne sglazit'*: *t'fu* is an imitation of spitting over one's left shoulder, to prevent *sglaz*, while *ne zglazit'* means literally 'do not let evil eye be put on me'.

This is a kind of *sglaz* caused by positive intentions. Of course, negative ones can result in *sglaz* just as well. As Katerina explained, *sglaz* can hit you everywhere and at any moment, without your being aware of it; it is 'like dirt that someone passing by splatters on your shoes'. You can be affected if a stranger in the street looks at you with anger or envy, loudly abuses you, or even silently wishes you harm. If you are unkind to other people and by arrogance or neglect offend them, they can cast *sglaz* on you with a wave of their anger, an élan of negatively charged intentionality unleashed in your direction. Or, as in the case with Marina, malevolence can be sweet-coated by flattery. You can receive *sglaz* if you happen to be a witness of violence or something else unpleasant. The moment of affliction does not need to be remembered, although it can be, as in the case with Marina. The evil eye does not start fatal transformations of your life immediately. It may affect your state of mind, your mood, or your current attitude to life. Anxiety, the beginning of depression, or irrational fears are possible manifestations of an effect of the evil eye.

According to Katerina, a simple *sglaz* can develop into *porcha* (noun from the verb *portit'*, to spoil). Or, more often, *porcha* can be inflicted on you by someone else, a relative, a neighbour, a co-worker. *Porcha*, another well-known term of affliction in Russian folk magic, is translated by English-speaking scholars of magic as 'spoiling' (Ivanits 1989, Ryan 1999); in peasant life, long before the revolution, it has been a popular designation of all sorts of harm. The range of misfortunes that Russian peasants attributed to *porcha* varied from crop failure, drought and the drying up of milk cows, to family discord, infertility and various illnesses (Ivanits 1989: 83). In her study of Russian folk beliefs Linda Ivanits noted that in Russian folk magic demonology was largely absent, although there were certain kinds of illnesses that were indeed attributed to demonic possession. Instead, the power of 'spoiling' was seen as an impersonal negative force from which the ill-wisher drew her power. This destructive force was then focused on a person, a grain field, or some enterprise, and resulted in a grave failure, illness or death.

According to my informants, *porcha* is sent with persistent, focussed intent to hurt you, by another person's pointed envy or resentment. Problems with male potency as well as female infertility might be diagnosed by a magus as the result of *porcha*, sent by an abandoned lover, or by a rival who has crossed your path, as in Marina's case. Rivals in love or business are often pointed out by magi as perpetrators of *porcha*, as are former spouses and in-laws. The latter are people who, by dint of their structural position, frequently compete for immediate physical space, literally the living-space (*zhilploshchad'*) of the home (square metres of residential space in apartments and summer houses (*dachas*) are a 'limited good' in Russian life and are often a source of impassioned hostilities).

When I probed Katerina about what *porcha* is, she answered through an extended metaphor. 'If you imagine a human being as an apple,' she said, 'and her biofield as the apple's flesh, then *porcha* is like a rotten or maggot-afflicted area of this apple.' So, *porcha* can be imagined as some kind of rot in the individual's non-physical body, that can be manifested to the eye of the magus as a darkened part of the client's aura, or as something exuding cold, or perhaps as a putrid smell, also purportedly sensed by the magus alone. In the presence of *porcha*, your life starts to suffer in a number of ways, felt as persistent bad luck, as failed relationships and failed projects, as accidents that come one after another, and, furthermore, as physical illnesses experienced by yourself and your family. I heard from several magi that patients with *porcha* were referred to them, unofficially, by biomedical institutions. These are patients with diffuse physical (and maybe mental and psychological) complaints for which biomedicine fails to identify causes.

Negativy like *sglaz* and *porcha* can go a long way to account for a multitude of problems. However, there are more terms in the vocabulary of magic. Two of these define more specific groups of misfortune, namely social isolation and failure to secure a partner. This, in Russia, may be a matter of considerable social stigma as well as a challenge to the individual's survival in a world where personal ties are the only existing safety networks. To be married, or to have been married once in the past, is an important part of the cultural definition of a social person. A woman, especially, who has never married is likely to be tacitly pitied and considered flawed and incomplete. Parents who fail to see their children (especially daughters) married may consider this as their major defeat in life. This is the background for the magical diagnosis known as 'the crown of celibacy' (*venets bezbrachiia*), a variety of a broader misfortune called 'the seal of loneliness' (*pechat' odinochestva*).

Nelli is an active, strong and smart woman in her early 30s. Having been educated as an engineer in a technical college, she managed to get a degree in economics and financial management through evening courses, and then found herself a wonderful job, versatile, challenging and well-paid. She has a lovely apartment and an intense social life, as her company, a franchise of a big Western firm, frequently arranges personnel get-togethers at bowling, bridge, and golf. She trains in aerobics, and enjoys enviably good health. The reason why she came to Inna was a persistent failure in the matters of the heart. 'I am respected and liked by my male colleagues, but when it comes to starting a romance, it is as if I become invisible. In my whole life, no one had as much as invited me out for dinner,' she told me in our conversation in Inna's kitchen. The diagnosis that Nelli received from Inna was 'the crown of celibacy'.

At the time I met Nelli, Inna had been working with her for two months. No serious suitors had yet turned up, but, according to Nelli, the ice had been broken, some attempts had been made. 'I don't have this damned crown any more, so I've got the green light. The problem now, for me, is to learn to manage it. I think they experience me as too eager'. According to both Inna and Nelli, the crown of celibacy has been removed, but they both agree that Nelli's behaviour with men is still to be honed. As Inna put it: 'The magical part is ready and done. What remains is the psychological part'.

'The crown of celibacy' has its aetiology in Russian folk tradition. The first and literal meaning of the word *venets* is a ritual crown which is part of the paraphernalia of the Russian Orthodox Church. It is used, among other solemn occasions, in the wedding ceremony, where crowns are held by the officiating priest over the heads of the wedded couple. *Venets* is also the Tsar's crown, and the coronation ceremony in pre-revolutionary Russia was called *venchaniie na tsarstvo*, with the meaning that the Tsar, God's chosen one, was wedded to Russia. In a similar way, nuns and priests are wedded to Christ when they take monastic vows. A woman who turns to a magus complaining that she cannot get a husband may hear, by way of a diagnosis, that she has 'a crown of celibacy', maybe as a result of some heinous deeds perpetrated by some of her ancestors many years ago.

A variety of this affliction, of a still graver character, is called 'a seal of loneliness' (*pechat' odinochestva*). It means that a person cannot develop any close relationships, cannot find anyone she can rely on, no one from whom to derive whatever joy sociality may bring: no relatives, friends, admirers, no significant others whatsoever. Be it as it may, both the seal of loneliness and the crown of celibacy are, in a way, the symptoms. In can happen that, in the course of interaction, the magus will uncover their initial cause. For example, these, and a number of other afflictions, can be triggered by the crimes or immoral deeds perpetrated by the victim's ancestors in the past.

This time, Tatiana's clients are Nina, a mother in her mid-thirties, and her eleven-year-old son, Serezha. Serezha is a lively, sturdy, healthy-looking boy, with an easy smile and a relaxed, self-assured manner.

He has a way with people, and he knows it. Tatiana starts small talk with him, and he replies eagerly and with a good deal of social competence. But his mother looks concerned. The boy is asked to go out of the room, and she tells Tatiana about her troubles. The boy is all right, but the mother has no authority with him whatsoever. He plays truant, he steals from his school-mates, he goes missing almost every day, and the mother has no way of checking where he spends his time. She found money that he had hidden away, and he would not tell her where it came from. He has a police record, having been detained several times. She feels that she has lost control, and she is terrified. This boy is all she has in her life.

The father left them several years ago. He was a brutal man, he drank and beat her, and she finally threw him out. Still, he continued to come and steal things from the apartment when she was away and it was Serezha who would let him in. The father worked as a driver of a street-cleaning truck, a vehicle that drives at night through the empty streets of the city, splashing them with water from the in-built hoses. One night he was driving very drunk, and he steered his truck right into a Mercedes car parked on the side of the street. The Mercedes belonged to a tough guy, and two men came to Serezha's father a couple of days later and said that 'they have put him on the counter': his life was ticking away, and if he didn't pay they would kill him. He told them that he did not have the money. He went to Nina and told her the story, begging her for a loan. She screamed at him that she had nothing to do with him anymore, that she would not have given him money even if she had it, and that he should get out. He left, cursing her.

Next week, one early morning when Nina and Serezha left their apartment on the way to work and school (Serezha was in second grade then), they saw the corpse of the father hanging from a hook in the ceiling right in front of their doorway.

Serezha seemed to take it with equanimity. He did not display any vehement emotions either on the spot or later. And he did not seem to miss his father or to talk about the incident. But after some time his whole personality changed. He was still the same loving son, but he was reticent about his whereabouts, and he was no longer obedient. He just stopped taking seriously whatever authority there was – neither his mother nor his teachers at school, not even the police. He was not rude or rebellious, he just seemed to have his own agenda that he did not share with anyone. And he was only eleven years old! Nina had strong fears about his future, and she had come to Tatiana to ask for help.

Serezha was called in again, Tatiana tried to talk with him, and he answered amiably, but noncomittally. She asked Nina if there was anyone among the older kin who had worked 'v organakh', a colloquial Russian expression meaning the structures of coercive power in the Soviet era, be it KGB or any of its many ramifications that had penetrated all work places in Soviet times. Nina confirmed that her ex-husband's grandfather had been a Red Army commander (komissar) working in the Ukraine during the 'de-kulakisation', the Bolshevik campaign in agricultural areas, when hidden stocks of grain were confiscated from wealthier peasants, the kulaks, who were then either killed or sent to Siberia.

Tatiana told Nina that here was a case of kinship curse that had been incurred on the grandfather by his victims, that was transmitted to the next generation to kill his son, and that was now at work destroying the last male in the lineage. Nina nodded comprehendingly, Serezha sat with glassy eyes, without reacting. The methods of treatment that Tatiana suggested were from the routine repertoire: rolling off with eggs, reading away with prayer, drinking water which had been charged with Tatiana's energy. When I met Nina several weeks later, however, this treatment did not seem to have brought about any changes in Serezha's behaviour.

A plain but healthy-looking woman in her early fifties turned to Tatiana complaining of a total lack of life energy. She had a good job as a book-keeper in a building firm, and a good husband who treated her well and brought his wages home. She had no precise reason to complain, except for the absence of any interest in life. 'Problems in your family life?' Tatiana opened up the conversation. 'No, my husband is very nice. He does not drink, he loves me, all he wants is to please me. He even brings me kasha in bed in the mornings, to make me happy, but ...' – 'You have a lover?' – 'No, I'm not like that! ...' 'You don't love you husband, do you?' asks Tatiana, looking at the woman probingly. 'No,' the woman answers calmly. 'And you don't have sex with him?' – 'No, I can't. I never particularly enjoyed it anyway, though in the beginning, many years ago now, I used to force myself... But it was never something I liked ... . I married him because he was so insistent, and because my mother used to nag at me that I was unmarried and close to thirty, she just could not let me be.' 'And you have never loved any man in your life?' The woman is strangely unperturbed, expressing no emotional reactions, a demeanour uncharacteristic of the clients of magi. A vague smile hovers over her lips, as if she is engaged in a social small-talk about the weather, not bringing her troubles to the magus in the hope of receiving help. 'No,' she admits calmly, 'I never loved anyone. I did have admirers, and even now, there are many men at work who give me looks, but I don't feel anything for any of them.' 'And you don't have children, do you?' 'No, we don't.' 'But what do you want from me?' 'Can't you do something that I would get some desire to live?' asks the woman, sounding unnaturally even, with the same faint and somewhat mocking smile on her lips.

Tatiana's face hardens perceptibly. She gives the woman a long, stern look. 'You have a kinship curse', she says. 'Do you know if your mother had someone she loved before she married your father?' No, the client doesn't know anything about it, and now her mother is dead and there is no way of asking. Her father was a middle-range Soviet official, much older than her mother, but he died when his daughter was still quite young, and she cannot remember anything about him or her parents' relationship. 'Well, that was the way it was,' Tatiana spells out her final judgement. 'Your mother had someone who loved her, and she was even pregnant by him. But she betrayed this love, had an abortion, and married an older man she did not love, for the sake of stability and well-being. The betrayal of her love and the murder of her love-child was what distorted the life programme of your kinship line. You don't know what love is, this is the form the kinship curse took on you, and this is what is bringing your lineage to an end. I can work with you, but only with your active cooperation. You must understand that love is the most important thing, and that you need to feel it, first and foremost towards your husband. But I warn you, it won't be easy!'

The woman is quiet, her facial expression unchanged. She says she will give it a thought and maybe see the receptionist and make an appointment. 'She won't come', Tatiana comments when the door closes behind the woman. 'This is a very difficult kinship curse, a hopeless case: her soul is dead, and so the lineage is winding up. She does not want anything, she does not love anyone, not even herself.

In fact, she does not want any treatment either. She came just because she has nothing better to do – she has no children to spend her money on ...'

In these two cases Tatiana has diagnosed 'kinship curse' (*rodovoie prokliatie*), a disturbance that affects the health and well-being of the victim and her loved ones, that comes from the past and steers the present into an inevitable future disaster, mortifying the very core of the self and programming it for destruction. Its roots seem so deep as to be at the limit of Tatiana's curing powers: when the soul is dead, Tatiana seems to imply, there is no recourse to healing. As far as Tatiana is concerned, the woman is already dead, a lost cause. By pointing out the late mother's betrayal of love and abortion as the cause of the kinship curse, Tatiana typically assumes the role of a moral arbiter, a lay equivalent to an Orthodox priest. But this is done more in the way of a casual comment: magi are not omnipotent, a sad truth known both to themselves and to their clients, and diagnosing a kinship curse is one way of saying that the case might well be beyond repair. Addictions, incurable diseases that strike young people, heavy and inexplicable accidents, and failures that affect all members of the family, and that tend to recur in similar patterns from generation to generation, hitting first parents and then all siblings, may be diagnosed as kinship curses. Often the magus traces the kinship curse to a certain ancestor, frequently one in the generation active during the early years of the revolution or during Stalin's reign of terror. This may be a grandparent who was known to turn people in, or to have worked in the KGB as an interrogator or an executor, or as a GULAG guard. The horror felt by the victims, and the hatred that they hurled at these people are understood to have disturbed the latter's 'energy-information structures', changing, as it were, the code of destiny, and causing troubles in the lives of their children and grandchildren. Or, as in the case above, it may be some other morally reprehensible action, the betrayal of an idealised romantic love and an abortion being two of the most usual. Or, it can be a more general human flaw, expressed in the inability to live up to moral expectations in parental and marital relationships, where responsibility and care are expected. Patients diagnosed with kinship curses can recall, in confirmation of the diagnosis, that someone in the family used to be exceptionally mean or quarrelsome, or that someone used to say to someone else in anger, 'Drop dead!' Cleavages in families in past generations do not disappear, but continue their destructive activity far into the future, scarring the lives of innocent descendants.

An interesting variety of affliction, pertaining to rather specific cases, is called 'demonic settlement', *demonicheskoiie podseleniie*. Like many of these terms, it has a strange and touching ring to it, carrying the mind back to times past and to recognisable everyday situations. *Podseleniie* is a term from the life of Russian communal flats, where several families lived in different rooms of one apartment, sharing kitchen and bathroom facilities. The communal apartment, an existential experience known to every Russian, was called by Svetlana Boym 'the cornerstone of the now disappearing Soviet civilization', 'a Soviet cultural unconscious' (see Boym [1994: 123] for a brilliant analysis of *kommunalki*). This specifically Soviet form of life, a hell of involuntary togetherness, was alleviated, but far from eradicated, by the massive residential construction programme of the later Khrushchev times (prefabricated apartment houses with tiny apartments, thin walls with no sound isolation, low ceilings, and dirty staircases, were popularly known as Khrushchoby, a composite from *Khrushchev's trushchoby*, Krushchev's slums. See also Boym 1994: 125). The word *podseleniie* evokes a situation where several families were squeezed into enforced proximity, and where additional, unwanted dwellers were put in by some external hostile power.

Demonicheskoie podseleniie can be translated approximately as 'the coercive settling of a demonic force'. The expression evokes the undesired presence of a strange agency, inserted into one's home against one's will, encroaching on a space that is already packed full. The diagnosis of 'demonic settlement' is given in cases when otherwise kind and peaceful persons tend to suddenly display quite opposite, threatening and destructive impulses that they themselves cannot control. One of the most usual manifestations of this affliction is a violent outbreak while in a state of intoxication, when an otherwise quiet and considerate person becomes a brute.

Lidiia and Anatolii are a young married couple, clients of Katerina. Lidiia comes from a Russian province, and graduated from the local Pedagogical Institute as a qualified school teacher. Anatolii lived with his mother in a tiny two-room apartment, a *Khrushchoba* as mentioned above. When he was dating Lidiia and it was clear that they had serious intentions, his mother told him at once that he should not even dream of moving his young bride in, much less registering her in the apartment, to get her a Moscow *propiska*. The *propiska* is the official registration at a certain address, that gives a person the right to live in a certain city, in this case Moscow, with all the entitlements this entails. To get registered in an apartment, one has to secure the formal agreement of the present tenants. Once the *propiska* is registered, the person has a legal right to a part of the apartment, which, in the case of future splits, such as divorce, leaves the previous dwellers with far less living space. Machinations around *propiska* are one of the causes of people becoming homeless, becoming a BOMZh, i.e. a person with no fixed abode, the most stigmatised status of a Russian citizen. Since living space in a big city, especially in one of the capitals, is a highly limited resource, the conflicts between the present and the prospective tenants, most often between young spouses and their in-laws, are one of the most usual sources of resentment.

Thus, when Anatolii married Lidiia, they had to find a place to live. Anatolii managed to rent a room in an apartment in another *Khrushchoba*. This room was tiny, dark and dirty, and consisted of a small shabby table that served as a desk as well as a dinner table, and a bed that the newly married were allowed to use. They lived in this room for about a year, Anatolii working as a bus driver, and Lidiia trying to find a job as a school teacher. This proved to be difficult, and she was turned down several times, precisely because she did not have the Moscow *propiska*. At some point Lidiia, a quiet and good-humoured person with a sunny and joyful disposition, started to be plagued by strange fits of hysteria. She would become furious over small things, and overcome with uncontrollable sobs of rage, beating herself against the floor, rocking and shaking so that she sometimes even hurt herself. Having calmed down, she would admit that her reactions were uncalled for, and she felt terribly sorry, but the attacks would start again for no apparent reason at all.

After much wandering from one *mag* to another, the couple finally found Katerina. After talking to them and consulting her cards, Katerina diagnosed a 'demonic settlement'. The hostile element, she said, came from the bed the young people were sleeping on. She saw that an old woman had died on this bed some time before the couple moved into the room. It was this woman, said Katerina, who had been the bearer of the demonic element before she died. To confirm her insight, she assigned the young people to carry out discreet investigations, to find out who had lived in their room before. The owner of the flat was unwilling to provide any information, but the neighbours confirmed that, indeed, there had been an old woman who had lived and died there. She had had a highly unpleasant temper (she was described by the neighbours as *skandal'naia starukha*, an old brawl-monger).

The first advice that Katerina gave the couple was to dispose of the bed as soon as possible, which they did after the owner reluctantly granted permission. Katerina made them understand that the act of throwing away the bed would not automatically free Lidiia from the demonic spirit, but that this was a necessary first measure before anything else could be undertaken. After a six-month course of treatment, Lidiia's fits stopped completely, according to Anatolii. Among other means there were the regular 'energy' treatments, the séances during which the demonic essence was actually banished. These were complemented by drinking water over which Katerina had read appropriate spells, reading away with prayer, regular visits to church, and morning and evening prayers that Lidiia was taught to read while lighting a candle in front of the Icon of the Mother of God that Katerina told them to buy and to hang on the wall, to protect the dwelling from the intrusion of any demonic elements in future.

An affliction that is a variety of demonic settlement, but that is even more difficult to deal with, is *oderzhaniie besami* – what could be translated, with some qualifications, as 'demonic possession'. The Russian words *'demon'* and *'bes'* are used as synonyms, although *'demon'* is perhaps an evil force greater and more awesome than *'bes'*. *Besy* (pl.) or *cherti* (sing. *chert*) are terms for a host of lesser evil beings of the Russian cultural imaginary; some of the *besy* or *cherti* can even be merry and mischievous, and in folk tales they play tricks against big bad guys on the side of the weak. This attitude is connoted by the diminutives *chertik, chertenok, besenok*, which can be used affectionately, for example, towards lively children (there is no corresponding diminutive for *demon*). So, *oderzhaniie besami* can be rendered as being possessed by diverse evil spirits, although in the context of magic those beings are seen as anything but harmless.

Scholars (e.g. Ryan 1999 and Ivanits 1989) agree that the main difference between Russian folk magic in pre-revolutionary times and Western witchcraft and sorcery was the lack of a philosophically grounded demonology. However, demons and the devil were not at all absent from folk beliefs. One of the most frequently encountered terms in their lexicon was *nechistaia sila* (or *nechist'*), 'unclean force(s)'. This term was a designation of the devil, but it also referred to all potentially harmful spirits in general, including *cherti* and *besy*. Popular belief attributed to sorcerers and witches the ability to send evil spirits to harm people. One form of this affliction was '*klikushestvo*', a disease that affected women and was attributed to demonic possession. It manifested itself as hysterical or epileptic attacks or violent outbursts, or as spectacular public fits of obscene behaviour (descriptions of *klikushestvo* and demonic possession remind one strongly of the symptoms of a psychoneurological disease called Tourette's syndrome, see., e.g. Sacks 1995).

In today's Russia, *klikushestvo* is not as common as it was in the old days (when, at times, it acquired epidemic proportions [Ivanits 1989]), but possession (*oderzhaniie*) does sometimes occur. It is tacitly agreed that magi are not powerful enough to deal with it. There is a small number of priests in the Russian Orthodox Church who are known to treat demonic possession. They usually live in monasteries and regularly offer services where they perform group exorcism. These services are reportedly highly crowded, dramatic, terrifying spectacles, believed to be dangerous for idle onlookers to witness, but visited by dozens of sufferers from all over Russia. The priests who can drive out demons are much in demand, and the Church turns a blind eye to their activities: even though healing is greatly discouraged by the Church, the tacit understanding is that its rare and chosen representatives are the only experts that can deal with it.

The following is a story of a woman suffering from demonic possession. At the time I met her she was a client of Katerina, and it was Katerina who asked her to talk to me. Liudmila, a stout, fresh-looking woman in her mid-fifties, spoke eagerly, clearly enjoying the opportunity of being able to tell her story.

Liudmila was born after the war, in a small village. She was a quiet, timid little girl. Her father had been killed in the war, and her mother brought her up alone. The mother was always tired, a gaunt, exhausted, austere woman, who never had a kind word for her daughter, although she was never outright mean. The only thing Liudmila liked when she was a child was to be around the village healer, an old woman, who lived in a nearby house. The girl liked to be stroked by her, to feel her hand on her head.

Liudmila grew up, moved to a small town, and got married. Her husband, who worked as a security guard at a military factory, did not drink or womanise; but he was a sullen, distant person, who liked to be left alone. She does not remember hearing a kind word from him either, she said, adding that this was certainly no reason for complaining about her husband. It was her mother-in-law who hated her deeply, even though they had never lived together; it was enough to be in the same town.

At some point Liudmila started to feel pains. 'How can I describe them? It's like a toothache you have, but it's all over the body, everywhere, inside, too. It prickles, itches and gnaws away at you. This is how it feels when the small imps and demons, all kinds of filth (*vsiakaia nechist'*), have crawled inside of you and start churning around. The pains were so strong that I wanted to wail. They put me in hospital and gave me a medical examination, but found nothing. I went to all sorts of *babki*, healers and fortune-tellers. They all told me that I had *porcha*, so strong that no one could dislodge it, and that it was someone who had 'worked' on me. I knew exactly who it was – my mother-in-law. But it was not just *porcha*, she sent the demons on me as well. I feel them inside me, they pinch me at night, and I wake up all bruised. Sometimes they rape me in my sleep, sometimes I see them as themselves, the demons, but other times they look like the men I know, who would never have had any truck with this kind of thing. In my waking life, I am not interested in sex at all. I stopped having sex with my husband when we had our second child. We now live in different rooms, and we almost never talk to each other. My children live separately, and it is only those healers that I can talk to. I have seen them all. The last one was a very powerful *mag*, an exorcist. He confirmed what I already knew, that I was possessed by demons, and promised to help. I don't know what he did, I always sat motionless, with my eyes closed. And these demons came out of me – they rolled me on the floor, they made me swear, roar, bark like a dog – and I have never used a word of foul language in my life!

Sometimes he put the mirror in front of me and commanded: 'You, demonic beings, show yourselves!' And they obeyed him, they showed their faces – it was not my face I saw in the mirror, but an animal smirk, fangs, and eyes burning with blue fire. They screamed, barked and roared! He drove them out, I felt better for a while, and then they would always come back. Finally, he said to me: 'That's it, we have done what we could. There are no demons in you, I have sealed off your demonic channel.'

'Yes, he said that, but I felt them, crawling and chasing about inside me, pinching and biting. I left him, and found Katerina, and it was the same story with her. It helped to begin with, I felt well for a week after the séance, but then it all came back again. Katerina did help me, she made my insides whole. My insides, I felt, had started to decompose, I felt I stank inside. Now I don't, but still the demons come back, they return more quickly now than before. I feel that Katerina is not strong enough to deal with them. She told me to go to church, but I can't. As soon as I enter the church, they start to break my bones, it hurts so much that I want to scream, to stand on all fours and weep like a wolf. My prayer does not reach [God], it is as if there is a barrier between me and Him. This is because the demonic channel is open, as soon as the demons are driven out, they come back again. I think it's time for me to die', she finished her story calmly.

What is worth noting here is that the client knows her diagnosis before the magi have had a chance to make it, that she literally feels the demons inside her body. She distinguishes *porcha*, generic 'spoiling' or rot, from demons making mischief inside her, even though she attributes both afflictions to the malevolent influence of her mother-in-law. The specialists confirm this diagnosis from the start. Both the client and the magi operate with two parts of her affliction: the demonic channel and the demons who enter Liudmila through this channel. Both sides agree that after the treatment sessions the demons leave. What they disagree on is what happens with the channel and with the demons afterwards. Katerina told me most definitely that Liudmila's demonic channel was sealed, that the demons were gone and were not coming back. She said, somewhat resentfully, that the woman was continuing to insist on their presence only because her affliction had become her identity, that made her meaningful to herself and gave her a story to tell to others. 'Look at her, she looks healthier than you or me!', Katerina remarked with distaste. Here, although the situation was conceptualised by the parties in the same terms, it was defined by them in different ways. For me, Liudmila's story can serve as an example of a failed treatment, although Katerina would never admit it.

'Demonic possession' is a cross-culturally recognised gloss of several indigenous ethnopsychologies that are parallel to what in Western psychiatry is known, for example, as schizophrenia, or as multiple personality disorder (see, e.g. Csordas 2002: 100–138). In general, various names of afflictions can be regarded as ethnopsychological terms, and magical treatment in Russia could lend itself to comparison with Western (post-Freudian) psychoanalysis. The most important similarity between the two lies in the understanding of self as a product of interpersonal processes. In this view, psychic life is composed of emotional configurations derived from relationships between self and others (Elliott 2002). One difference is that, for those who practise magic in Russia, it is not only the psyche that is so constituted, but, moreover, the physical bodies of self and her significant others, as well as material and situational configurations of her life. Comparison between indigenous healing and Western psychoanalysis was at the core of the approach taken by Lévi-Strauss in 'The Effectiveness of Symbols' (1963), an essay that I shall return to below. In this book, however, I consciously chose to forego any systematic comparison between Russian magic and Western psychoanalysis, guided by Kleinman's warning against 'professional transformations' of the subjectivities of suffering and practices of coping when we interpret them, in psychoanalytic terms, as 'the symbolization of dynamic conflicts in the interior of the self' (Kleinman 1995: 96). Although the activities of magi do, to a degree, remind one of those of Western analysts (and I shall briefly return to this point in a later chapter), the whole language of psychoanalysis hinges on notions of pathology and normality that are too closely connected with the normative Western models of an autonomous, wholly individuated self, not fully applicable to the realities of Russia.

Names given to afflictions can be adduced. Some belong to a common stock, shared among magi, and known to lay people. There are also idiosyncratic terms that individual magi coin for their own practice, perhaps to suit specific cases. Recall Misha, with his 'little scarf of bad luck' (*sharfik nevezeniia*) that caused him so much chagrin. Another client was said to be covered by a strange tangle of woollen threads or hairs, visible only to the magus, but encumbering the person in all his movements so that his life became unbearable. Common to all instances of magical treatment is that the first – and the most important – step in this therapeutic interaction is to give an affliction a name. I shall now consider this act of naming as semiosis – the process of generating signs in the consciousness that have the potential of changing the patient's picture of the world and of the self.

Terms of affliction as icons and indexes

It is an accepted premise in medical anthropology that giving an affliction a name is the first step to curing. In his classical essay 'The Effectiveness of Symbols', Lévi-Strauss (1963) compared shamanic healing with Western psychoanalysis, to show that the same mechanism of cure was involved in these both processes. The pains of the patient, be it physical pains of the Cuna woman in difficult childbirth (analysed in the essay), or psychosomatic pains of a modern Western urbanite, were named, personified, and set into a meaningful narrative structure (Lévi-Strauss called it 'mythology'). In both cases, the patient was provided with the language with which inchoate pains could be expressed; 'conflicts and resistances' (p. 198) that had been torturing the sick person were brought from her unconscious on the conscious level.

Even Lévi-Strauss, however, was aware that such attempts to interpret native healing techniques would remain meaningless unless we can explain 'how specific psychological representations are invoked to combat equally specific ... disturbances' (p. 191). More recently, Csordas (1997a) pointed out that healing efficacy is to be sought in the particularities of healing interactions. Following Csordas, let us see how in Russian magic phenomenological changes could be achieved by the semiotic ones. To that end, let us look at the process of semiosis unfolding in some of the cases described above.

The concepts of the crown of celibacy, *sglaz*, *porcha*, kinship curse, or demonic beings can be regarded as Representamina. Their Objects are not in the nature of physical objects or concrete events. Instead, it is a diffuse state of misfortune, loneliness, and the feeling of powerlessness to shape one's life in a socially acceptable way that is at stake here. However, while the Object in these cases may be undefined, in the diagnostic interactions it receives a concrete Representamen. It is offered to the patient as a concept, and it stays with her as a perceptual 'image-in-consciousness'. The latter concept was used by Csordas (1997b) to account for the healing effect that images in consciousness have for American Catholic Charismatics. As Csordas observes, an Interpretant here is not 'another sign' that represents, but the whole experience of the situation or problem indicated, or 'indexed' by this sign. The term of affliction becomes, in Csordas's words, 'a function of embodiment, ... the pragmatic engagement in the world' (p. 85).

But, as signs, the Russian magical terms of affliction are rather pragmatically singular: they are not 'imaginal performances' described by Csordas for the American Charismatics. Instead, they are exclusively object-images of disturbances. For the patients, part of their meaning is constituted by the idea of causal, or existential, connection, as it is in the nature of indexical signs. Moreover, they are introduced to patients with one purpose only: to be removed as soon as possible by the magus's skills.

By presenting a missing link in the chain of causation, in diagnosis, the magus introduces into the patient's consciousness and life-world a concrete and recognisable object. Now it is this object that is seen to cause the trouble. In the same way that a blowing wind causes a weather-cock to turn, or the feet of a walking person cause his footsteps to make impressions in the sand (textbook examples of indexical signs), so the imaginary crown of celibacy causes Nelli's loneliness and inability to find a partner; and the 'spoiling' or 'rot' in the living essence of a person's 'bio-field' causes her strength to drain away so that she is prevented from enjoying a full-fledged life.

Indexicality, however, is only one facet of these signs. The Objects as images-in-consciousness are iconic representations of actually existent cultural 'objects' (from real life or cultural imaginary). They work through visual similarity with their worldly prototypes. Thus, Nelli talks about 'that damned crown' that is now taken away, presumably having in mind a visual image of a church crown used for wedding together man and wife. Likewise, the general idea of *porcha* goes some way to concretise the 'inchoate pains', as in Lévi-Strauss's analysis discussed above. In specific interactions with the magi this rather vague notion takes on concrete dimensions, giving shape to a certain, however incipient, narrative, or to what Lévi-Strauss calls 'mythology'. Comparing the Cuna healing chant and the interaction in psychoanalysis, Lévi-Strauss mentions that the only difference is in the nature of the mythology offered: in the first case it is a shared cultural mythology, while in the second case it is a personal one. In Russian magic, the situation is somewhere in between: what is offered to a patient is his or her personal mythology, embracing several generations of kin, and spelled out in shared terms. Thus, after speaking with the magus, people might visualise the healthy flesh of their 'thin body', covered with 'dirt' that is the essence of someone's intention to hurt, and even rotting as the result of this evil intention.

The terms of affliction, as signs, are symbolic and iconic with respect to the external work of culture, the repository of both images and language, and indexical with respect to the inner world of the patients; e.g. the crown of celibacy indexes loneliness even as it causally produces it. When these objects are removed from the patient's horizon of possibilities, their potentiality to cause misfortune also disappears, which may lead to an alleviation of the misfortune itself.

Evocation and the signs that present

Here, in accordance with Singer, 'emotional and energetic interpretants of iconic and indexical signs are not simply further signs but the interpreter's experience of qualities and interactions' (1980: 501). They are less texts to be deciphered, more tasks to be performed, actions to be accomplished, pragmatic interventions that modify first the field of perception, and then, possibly, the social situation. The conscious subjects are not only the readers of signs, but first and foremost 'pragmatically engaged body subjects bound to the world through their projects, which are not just interpretative projects.' (Innis 1994: 7). The Interpretants are more visual than discursive forms, grasped by the patient integrally. The semantics they are generated through is that which can be referred to as presentational semiosis (from Langer's [1986] 'presentational symbolism'), to be distinguished from the discursive symbolism of language proper.

These signs evoke and present due to their virtuality. Virtuality, an intriguing quality of magic, performance and modern computer entertainment, is defined as 'being such in essence though not formally recognised or admitted' (Oxford English Dictionary). In the contexts of computer-generated virtual reality, it means that the subject experiences reality as real, to all intents and purposes, whereas it is perhaps not recognised as such, 'objectively', by an outside observer. In magic rituals, Kapferer defined virtuality as 'constitutive and generative of practice, ... backgrounding and indexing this practice' (1997: 179–180). As he further details, 'virtuality is integral to the lived-in world but not subject to indeterminacies of its processes within forces of actuality' (ibid.).

Through their virtuality, the terms of affliction as signs redefine the client's world, giving it meaning, giving its misfortunes a cause, and presenting a concrete object to get rid of. By virtue of their dual mode of signification – iconic with respect to the external cultural world, the repository of both images and language; and indexical with respect to the inner world of the patient, since the signs are taken virtually to produce the patient's condition – the semiotic operations of magical diagnostic, and the ensuing treatment, are pragmatic in the sense envisaged by Peirce. 'Pragmaticism consists in holding that the purport of any concept is in its conceived bearing upon our conduct' (Peirce 1958: 221). Pragmaticism, for Peirce, expresses the relationship of signs and their processes to some definite human purpose. The purport of the magical terms of affliction, used in diagnostics as the first step of any treatment, is in its bearing upon the conduct of life.

The means of treatment

When describing the Centaur centre I have already given a glimpse of the magus's working premises, and of the instruments she used. Let us look more closely at Katerina's room, and at her tools and methods. Even though she moved several times during the years I knew her, thrown out by the flat owners without prior notice, in each new place Katerina took care to recreate her working room to look the same. The light in this room was always subdued, a window covered by a heavy velvet curtain. There was a low table and two deep armchairs either side of it, so that the magus and the client would sit facing each other during the initial conversation. That lasted an hour at the first meeting, and became shorter at the repeated visits that were mostly devoted to 'treatment' proper. On the table, there were several small icons, a Bible, a Russian Orthodox prayer book, and a slender silver candlestick with thin wax candles of the type that one buys in church. Also in the room was a chair put in the centre of a pentagram within a circle drawn in chalk on the floor, on which the patient sat during treatment, her eyes closed. This pentagram was Katerina's idiosyncrasy, the reflection of her interest in the Western occultism; I have never seen it in any other magus's consulting rooms. A tape recorder, playing New Age music during the treatment, completed the picture.

Prayer books, candlesticks and Russian Orthodox icons were always plentiful in magi's working rooms. This ubiquitous presence of icons was explained to me by a young, tough, and pointedly secularised healer who otherwise tried to forego all references to the Church and confided that the roots of her practice lay in Reiki healing. 'I don't care about Russian Orthodoxy,' she said, pointing to the latter-day, kitschy creations on the walls of her small apartment, as if apologising to me for their presence there. 'People need images of love and kindness – things that they can immediately relate to, and this is what icons are.'

This usage of the church symbolism for healing, already mentioned in the previous chapter, deserves a brief discussion. Anthropologist Sergei Oushakine, in his work on post-Soviet identity construction, introduced the notion of 'aphasia' – the absence of symbolic language in which the self and subjectivity can be spelled out (2000). There are no 'codes with which to dissect the knots of reality, ... no symbols to provide the mechanisms for production of subjectivity and agency' (p. 1005). This, according to Oushakine, leads to 'hermeneutic paralysis', the dissolution of subjectivity and the loss of self. One of the reasons for this, suggests Oushakine, is the 'absence of the field of cultural production' in the post-Soviet public sphere. To qualify this idea for the purposes of this book, I would say that what is lacking is perhaps some few well-defined and widely accepted 'fields of cultural production', of the type provided in Soviet times by the official 'kul'tura', with which people communed by reading Pushkin or by visiting the Tret'iakov Gallery. In contemporary Russia, there are certainly numbers of smaller, fuzzier and more problematic fields that offer signifiers to shape the post-Soviet experience. Their legitimacy and appeal are never finally established nor unproblematically shared, and therefore they easily transform and disappear. The Russian Orthodox Church is one of these fields, with a strong claim to cultural domination and moral legitimacy. One of its legitimation strategies is the move back into the past, or, as Oushakine puts it, 'regression into the previous cultural styles', a tendency that is comparable with what I referred to as 'legitimation by tradition'. It is therefore no wonder that magic relies so heavily on the Church for the relevant symbols.

But let us come back to the therapeutic interaction between the magus and the client. The first encounter, where the problem to be treated is initially presented, largely defines the patient's attitude to the magus (and possibly determines the success of the entire treatment). The way a magus listens to her clients is an essential part of her art. It is important for the client to have a chance to tell her story, to be listened to in a sympathetic but not too indulgent way, encouraging, but not too pitying. The magus should confirm the patient both as sufferer and agent, clarifying her vision to discern whatever delusions may blur it, but not maligning too much those who seem for the moment to be the source of her problems. The magus should not ask too many questions, lest the client start to doubt her clairvoyant abilities. Some clients who come to a specialist for the first time are fond of challenging the magus, setting tests for her, for example showing her a photograph of a person and asking for information.

Some magi claim to see all the client's problems right from the start, rendering the client's narrative superfluous. This saves magi's time, which is important in a context like that of 'Centaur', when magi's time is money, but it is not necessarily the best for the clients, who tend to consider such short shrift as coldness and lack of attention. Thus, the first conversation must be a fine balance between saying too much and too little. Usually, a good first consultation is a dialogue, reminiscent of the interaction between diviners and their clients described by Whyte for Eastern Uganda (1998). The props of this dialogical interaction, however, are individual. Katerina, for example, uses her tarot cards, as if checking what the client discloses against what the cards show and what she herself sees. Along the course of the narration, she asks questions, makes comments, and offers details. As in the case of the Ugandan diviners, it was important for Katerina that her hints were confirmed. If the client sees her rejoinders as cues for further disclosures, this first interaction can be meaningful for both and fruitful for the client in sorting out the conundrums of her life.

After this dialogue, the diagnosis is set in the terms discussed above, and treatment is defined. This treatment consists of a limited number of basic elements. Often, the magus provides the client with the requisite spells for specific life situations, from securing the benevolence of one's boss, to getting rid of an eye cataract or a tumour, to diverting a husband from alcohol or drugs, or ensuring a good growth of the vegetable garden at the dacha. The spells are read by the magus herself, over water that the client is asked to drink; or the client is instructed to read them herself, for example over the vodka that her husband will drink at dinner, or over the water she will use to water her garden. Sometimes this method is simplified, and the spell part is omitted. Instead, the magus charges the water (in a bottle) with her energy, and the patient is advised to drink it, and to use it to wash her hands and face, or ailing parts of the body.

One method that is used by many magi is called '*otchityvaniie molitvoi*', literally, reading away the negative energy with a prayer. The magus reads from a prayer book, in a loud, steady voice, for a lengthy period of time, up to twenty minutes. The words of the prayer, written in archaic language no longer used in everyday speech, are hardly discernible, and the sound of the magus's voice pours over the patient like a flood of purifying water.

Another widely used method, used more by those who refer to the Russian village tradition, is 'rolling off' (the negative energies) with an egg. The idea of this treatment is that the egg absorbs the negative energies drawn from the body of the patient. After the treatment, the magus might give the egg to the patient to feel the added weight of the '*negativy*' that had been sucked into the egg. The magus cracks the egg open and pours its contents into a glass of water, pointing out the impurities, coagulations, unevenness in texture, that, for the patient, visually represent the negatives extracted from her body.

Both methods are striking examples of indexical action. The patient feels the purifying essence of the words of the payer, whose 'meaning', discursively conceived, she does not understand. Nor is there any obvious discursive meaning in the operations with the egg.

Instead, it is understood to act pragmatically, like a vacuum cleaner. When the egg is cracked open, the patient sees the harmful intrusions, taken shape, disappear – the healer pours the contents of the egg into a glass, where the patient can contemplate them before they disappear in the sink. In these operations the 'negatives' are first presented verbally as something material, something alien to the body, and are then extracted as such, as 'matter out of place', pragmatically rather than symbolically. It should be noted, however, that in both of these cases, the choice of the tool for this practical action is not fortuitous. The words of the prayer books are repositories of power and purity by virtue of their being archaic, their belonging to the ancient Russian tradition. The egg is a 'natural symbol' of purity of nature, associated with germinating life that will grow under the warm shelter of the mother's body. As if to make this message more explicit, some magi make the acquisition of eggs for this purpose a veritable pilgrimage, telling their clients not to buy eggs at the supermarket or at a grocery store round the corner, but sending them instead to remote village markets, where transactions are not contaminated by the abstract economic structures of new capitalism, but are formed face to face with the individual producers whose hens laid the eggs that very morning.

The pantomime of healing

These methods are optional and complement the core, hand healing. With Katerina, the patient sits on the chair, her back straight, her palms on her lap. Katerina stands facing the patient, some three metres away. She puts on the music, lights the candles on the side table, and commands the person to close her eyes. Concentrating her gaze on the person, she creates with her hands the 'energy-information field' of the perfect being, as she sees it. Her movements can be likened to those of a sculptor moulding clay; or a weaver creating a tapestry from threads and ribbons; or a florist pulling, drawing and smoothing leaves, petals and stalks to shape an artistic design. These are all similes that give a vague idea of her movements, but do not describe them with any precision. As with other kinds of pantomime, it is easier to describe the virtual worlds we become witnesses to through the movements of the mime, than the movements themselves. Katerina's movements give life to a plethora of channels, vibrating flows that penetrate the oval-shaped field surrounding the person like blood arteries. These channels connect the human being with the higher realms, the realms to which the healer's stretched fingers sometimes point, and from which she draws the material she uses in her creation process. When these channels are blocked, or when some foreign matter clogs and litters the space that surrounds the body, then the individual is in trouble. It is this 'matter out of place' that Katerina plucks, pulls and lures out of the 'thin body' with her infinitely expressive hands, casting it out beyond the confines of the individual's immediate vital sphere.

Other examples of hand healing are presented in Chapter 5. Here, it will suffice to say that all the healing that I observed was a masterful pantomime, evoking the reality of the treated body that is never identical for two different healers nor two different patients, but that always displays the same essential ontological design. The process described above for Katerina differs somewhat from that employed by the healers who work with the reality of the body conceived of in conventional terms. Since they treat diseases indexed by symptoms, and understood to be caused by the chemical or mechanical dysfunctions of the inner biological machinery, their hands-on work proceeds in a much closer contact with the body proper. They might put the palms of their hands on the surface of the body under which the organ diagnosed as afflicted is located. Recall that many healers also report having inner vision, and they not only 'feel' the ill organs through their energy (*energeticheski*), but they also see it as if the body itself were transparent, as if by X-ray. With many healers, patients report a sensation of directed and intense warmth or heat, or electric-like discharges as if from an electrode, which emanate from the healer's hands and penetrate the body. When I was myself under treatment, I commented on this heat radiating from the hands of the healer; she put her hand on mine and commanded me: 'Feel!' Her hand itself was of a normal temperature, rather cool than warm; but, put back on the surface of the body where she diagnosed the afflicted organ, this penetrating heat was physically perceptible deep inside the body. Other healers work with a 'contactless' method, but move their hands over the patient's body, five to ten centimetres away from it, as if they were dealing with a liquid or other viscous medium that they physically put into motion as they deem appropriate.

This gestural mimesis of an imagined and embodied disorder is a pantomimic performance where the healer mends, or straightens up, with her hands whatever is conceived to be wrong – biomedically, energy-wise, or in terms of flows that connect the human being with the cosmos and make up the vital essence of her body. In all these cases, diagnosis is made in the indexical mood. It may be conceived biomedically, saying that pain in the lower abdomen is caused, say, by prostate inflammation, which is further understood as certain physical disturbances of tissues or organs. Or, it may be explained in terms of energy, when blockages of energy flows in channels or chunks of hostile negative energies cause illnesses and other misfortunes. During the pantomime of healing, these pictures are projected before the healer's mind's eye, and are presented to her consciousness as clearly delineated three-dimensional images (this, I suppose, is what the healers mean when they say that they 'see' these pictures).

The healer then treats these ill organs or these jumbled energy fields pragmatically, re-presenting, through pantomimic movements, what she would have done were they to materialise as flows, or were she to have had the possibility of actually touching them with her hands. In this silent, gestural performance, these images in consciousness interact with the healer's bodily movements and create a complex virtual reality, the process that for the healer emerges with pragmatic, physical concreteness.

This could be compared with the classical case of the shaman Quesalid, described by Lévi-Strauss in 'The Sorcerer and His Magic'(1963), where the shaman uses sleight of hand to offer the patient the material embodiment of her illness. Here, however, the crucial difference (and the fact that undermines conventional anthropological ways of explanation) is that, more often than not, the patient does not see anything of the spectacle. For example, Katerina's patients may have visions of varying clarity and detail, physical or emotional sensations such as heat or cold, sorrow or elation. Sometimes, tears silently roll down patients' cheeks, or they might break into uncontrollable sobs. These perceptions are important feedback for healers, they are keenly awaited, and the clients' comments and narratives about them are highly appreciated. If the client feels nothing at all (which also happens), or if she refuses to report her sensations under treatment, the magus becomes thoroughly disappointed, and the treatment may be soon terminated.

However, I could never elicit from any healer a direct or clear-cut connection between these patients' reactions and the healers' own pantomimic actions. It appears that healers are sole inhabitants of the universes created by their pantomimes (shared, as an exception, by the anthropologist or by a close relative). Katerina, for one, worked in a dark room, alone with the patient. In other cases, these movements are performed in broad daylight, in the presence of relatives, assistants and other patients awaiting their turn (as will be described in Chapter 5); sometimes these spectators pay attention, while at others they do not seem to bother and go about their own business. Therefore, speculations pertaining to possible connections between consciousness and matter must concern only the consciousness of the healer herself. My sense is that it is her own conviction in her powers that matters most in this process.

In conclusion, let me once again return to the comparison of magic healing in Russia and Western psychoanalysis. As indicated before, the first phases of the séance are based on letting the patient talk, while offering him or her names for their diffuse experience of misery. In the terms of Saussurian semiotics, espoused, for example, by Oushakine (2000) (in explaining the affliction of the society as a whole), the signifiers drawn from the cultural styles of the past offer meaning to the individual experience. The roots of this exercise can be traced to the tradition of *hermeneutics*, the search for meaning through interpretation of texts, the basis for confessional practices at the heart of psychoanalysis. But, as Kharkhordin suggested, subjectifying practices in Russia were based on a different technology, that of *homiletics*, where preaching led to a direct experience, bypassing meaning. (1999: 258, n. 93). In this way of knowing, meaning was revealed indexically, as a direct embodied knowledge, rather than symbolically, by matching the signifiers and the signifieds. It is the emphasis on this indexical mode of transformation that distinguishes a magic séance in Russia from its counterpart in Western psychotherapy.

Chapter 3
Magic as Management of Emotions

Let us return to Centaur and to Tatiana's consulting room, and take a closer look at the initial verbal exchange that starts the therapeutic process. Her clients in the instance I describe are a middle-class, rather wealthy-looking woman in her late forties and her son, in his late teens, handsome, well-groomed, well-dressed, and well-demeanoured. During the session he is mostly silent, smiling wearily and nodding slightly, to confirm what his mother is saying. According to his mother, everything, until just recently, has seemed to turn out very well for him. He had been admitted into a prestigious college, where he studied well, but he has recently quit his studies. Girls like him, he used to be a fine athlete, and now there is nothing specifically wrong with his health, but ... he does not want to live.

'Let's ask Tolia himself,' suggests Tatiana.

The boy speaks reluctantly, in a low voice, and with effort. 'I don't know what it is. I don't have any desire or strength to do anything. My body just refuses to obey me. And I am in pain, all the time. It's not physical pain, but some strange pain of the soul ...'

'Is there any bad company around him?' asks Tatiana. 'No, there used to be, but we took him away, we even had to move to another area of Moscow. He has no friends now, only a girl who he used to go out with, until recently. I suspect it is *porcha*,' the mother answers.

I see Tatiana twitch with impatience – she clearly does not like clients to come to her with ready-made diagnoses. 'Let's examine him,' she says. 'Come and stand here. Relax, close your eyes, and don't think about anything.'

As she moves her hands along the boy's body, her face becomes distorted with pain. 'I saw it from the start,' she says. 'Immediately as you came in, I saw this *porcha* on you. Your field is otherwise very weak – you have no protection – and this spot here, this area, feels like freezing cold.'

'That is exactly what I thought,' exclaims the mother, 'I knew he had *porcha*, and I even know who brought it on him ...'

'Who brought it on him is irrelevant,' interrupts Tatiana sternly, 'That person will be duly punished – you don't want to know those horrible things that will happen to this person. But this is not the point now. What we need to do is to remove the *porcha*. This is a well-advanced case, so it will take time. At least three séances. Reading off with a prayer, cleansing the aura. Let's start now.'

The mother insists on discussing who the agent of the *porcha* was. 'I know who it is,' she continues. 'It is his former girlfriend and her mother. They wanted to keep him so badly that they would've stopped short at nothing. What shall we do with them?'

Tatiana replies with well-monitored irritation, aptly conveying that she is cross, but restrains herself, taking on the role of a wise peacemaker. 'Go to church and light a candle for their health,' she says, 'Don't harbour bad feelings against them [*ne derzhite na nikh zla*]. All the black magic they have worked will return to haunt them, many times over. You should feel really sorry for them, how they will be tortured now [after this treatment], how they will writhe and roast [*krutit' da podzharivat*]' [these are the punishments that await the sinner in the Russian Orthodox Hell, according to the popular religious imagination.] 'By the way,' Tatiana continues, now suddenly talking about Tolia's mother in the third person, 'Not only son, but mother as well is afflicted by *porcha*. But the mother is stronger, so the consequences are not as bad. Your boy is a sensitive person' – now she addresses the mother directly – 'Strong as steel, but sensitive. Now I can see that this *porcha* has been cast on the entire family.'

The mother eagerly takes up the cue: 'Yes, there are huge problems also with my elder son. He married a divorced woman with a child, and she twists and turns him every way she wants [*vertit im kak khochet*]. He dressed her up from top to toe, she is wallowing in money, while he has completely forgotten about his mother ...'

Tolia suddenly raises his voice. 'She must be the one who set the *porcha*,' he suggests vehemently, in a manner that strikingly contrasts with the listless indifference he displayed earlier. But Tatiana abruptly shuts him up, as if banishing the whole subject from their conversation. 'He must be read away with prayer [*otchitat' molitvoi*], and he must be rolled off with an egg [*otkatat' iaitsom*],' she sums up, clearly showing her clients that she wants to be no part of this foe-finding intelligence raid. 'Now I see that we won't make it in three séances. Six times are more like it – I will alternate reading with egg-rolling. Sign up for an appointment [for the next visit] with the cashier [*zapishites' v kasse*],' she ends, giving them to understand that their time is up.

Absent anger

This brief episode captures themes that are played out, in varying ways, in many interactions between magi and their clients. First of all, it evokes the notion of 'therapeutic unit', once introduced by Arthur Kleinman (1980). It reminds us that, in many cultural contexts, illness is far from an individual affair; when it strikes, it affects a family as a 'body social' that involves the living and sometimes even the dead (as in the cases of 'kinship curse' discussed in the previous chapter, c.f. Whyte 1998). The affliction is located not only in the physical body of the patient but, as well, in the affective ties, expected and failed commitments, contested moral obligations that entangle its members, that both bind people together and tear them apart (this corresponds with the way psychotherapy views the self as constituted through emotional impulses and interpersonal relations). The person is seldom afflicted as a separate individual (notwithstanding the cases of the 'seal of loneliness', where the absence of social ties is a grave problem per se); and it is these bonds that also become loci of healing, what Csordas once called 'a locus of efficacy' (1997b).

This episode also shows that the seedbed of magic is the field of affects and the strong emotions invested in these bonds. It is the force of these affects that gives people strength to push and pull on one another, that underlies the vibrant intensity of human interactions, but that also make them vulnerable. It also demonstrates that part of the work of a magus is that of a preacher – that of moral arbitration and direction – as well as that of a psychoanalyst – that of management, if not outright manipulation, of these emotions and passions.

The idea that nonbiomedical healing involves changes in the structures of subjectivity is deep at the core of medical anthropology. It is implied in the view of illness as a 'syndrome of experience', 'a set of words and feelings that "run together" for members of a society' (Good 1977: 27). The main quest of medical anthropology, therefore, has long been to understand these experiences of illness in relation to local social worlds. It is also an accepted premise in medical anthropology that symbolic practices are central to the construction of illness experiences and to the production of the life-worlds of patients and their families. Starting from the work of Lévi-Strauss, the activities of native healers were analysed in terms of the new symbolic language that they provide to the patients in order to render their pain meaningful. This can work to alleviate this pain, because symbols are embodied, connecting social and physical realities. The work on embodiment, pioneered in anthropology by Thomas Csordas, pointed at inextricable connections between symbolic processes and bodily changes. In counterposition with more cognitivist views of culture as located in 'mind', that is in knowledge, symbols and meaning, the notion of embodiment pointed at the body as a generative source of culture, orientation and experience. Theorising embodiment also offered the potential to transcend the previous split in the study of emotions between the essentialists (those who reduced emotions to universal biological processes) and the constructivists (those who insisted that emotions were culturally constructed and could be studied only through their discursive expressions). In the embodiment literature, the embodied character of emotions was seen as precisely what made them social: as Lyon and Barbalet wrote, 'emotion is ... the means whereby human bodies achieve social ontology through which institutions are created: it is active in making its social world' (1994: 57). According to Kleinman's formulation, culture could be seen as patterning the relations between 'physiology, feeling, self-concept, body image, interpersonal communication, practical action, ideology, and the relationships of power' (1995: 179).

The involvement of the embodied self in the world, through emotions, is what magic deals with, in Russia as elsewhere. To understand how the changes that magic treatment purports to achieve can come to pass, a brief discussion of the terms pertaining to the study of emotions might be necessary. If magic is aimed at altering subjectivity and the self, and if self is in its essence emotional, then what remains is to account for the concept of 'emotions'. Most scholars agree that 'emotion' is both feeling and meaning (see Leavitt 1996; Milton 2002): both uniquely experienced, and accounted for in terms of the local culture. To avoid confusion, let me define the terms as I use them here (which does not necessarily coincide with the ways these terms are used by other authors). I understand 'affect' as a movement of the self in its engagement with the world, one of the expressions of the 'effort' mentioned by Csordas (1997b). Affect can be forceful, leading to violent actions, or, it can be latent and 'soft', a mere passing sensation with no exit to semiosis. Passions are instances of affect, but affects are broader than passions.

What I shall here call 'emotion' is affect already involved in the semiosis of social life, feeling which is imparted meaning by culture, reflexivity added to effort. Emotions in my usage here are both embodied or physically felt, *and* cognized, reflected upon in social categories. If affects (in my usage of the term) can be conceived of as presocial and private states, emotions are always elicited in specific contexts of social interaction. What emotions are about are forms of relations that exist between the subject and the world; they are always about the logic of engagement in social contexts, the logic that is governed by, and that can be read as, the linguistic codes and concepts of 'feeling-meaning states' (Leavitt 1996).

Instead of looking at biochemical or 'mechanical' states of the body (as, for example, in Ekman [1984]), Myers (1998) suggests turning to what he calls 'logical forms' of specific emotional states. These logical forms are structures of relationship between the individual and the circumstances that particular culture renders evident through discourses, socialisation rules and cultural scripts (Wierzbicka 1994). There are certain situations that prompt certain feelings, or trigger certain reactions and actions (or, for that matter, prohibit them), and so constitute the ways in which the individual interprets these situations. These ways are shared within a culture, but they are also idiosyncratic to individuals and groups. This way of seeing emotions allows for the fact that, even within the same culture, different individuals, depending on their social background and psychological make-up, might respond to shame, fear and joy in somewhat differing ways, although the emotion terms connected with these situations and the responses they elicit may be recognised and thus culturally shared.

The notion of logical forms of emotions, according to Myers, allows us to reconsider the 'representational view of emotions', whereby a signifier – an emotion term – corresponds to a signified conceived as a neurobiological state. Instead, he proposes to use the Peircian triad of Object, Representamen and Interpretant, to trace a connection between the logic of involvement, cultural prescriptions for reactions, and the lexemes – emotion terms – that may or may not be offered by the language. From this viewpoint, the 'emotives' offered by language – 'joy', 'anger', 'guilt' in English, *fago* in Ifaluk, *malu* in Indonesian, *obida* and *liubov'* in Russian – are, as all linguistic units, signs or Representamina. Their Object is a complex state of situational involvement with which culture-bearers identify the emotive in any concrete situation. The Interpretant is the sign that is formed in the consciousness of the Interpreter by resorting to cultural resources: the state/mood/feeling that is occasioned and the ensuing reactions. The Interpretant is formed through the socialised cognizance of the emotion terms and it presupposes strategic cultural knowledge that allows the subject to access the situation, to choose between its possible interpretations, and between possible courses of action. Since the Object in this semiosis is always situational, the Interpretants are ambiguous even within one culture, as always where affects are involved. They may depend on the cultural understandings surrounding the emotion terms, which may differ for different social groups within one culture, and they are contingent on the individual's biographic, psychological and biological idiosyncrasies.

This model allows for the analysis of pragmatic meaning of the emotion terms – not as fixed referents, but as diffuse incentives for action. It allows for ambiguity and ambivalence, and it also allows one to take account of dissimulation, faking, and intersubjective manipulation of emotional responses. This is often the case with magic as a cultural mode of managing emotional moods and motivations, the forces that animate the dynamics of engagement that is the self. This model also allows one to bring the body more firmly into the picture, because the Interpretant may eschew language altogether, being instead a totally embodied state of being, a presentation that defies any representation. This latter can be exemplified by the bodily feeling of elation beyond words that is part of the emotion of joy or of romantic passion. Or, it can be the shock of abasement with no Object identifiable, terminating the chain of signification and expressed in bodily sensations of pure pain, with no contingent meaning, as in 'phobias' or 'somatic problems', the predicaments which are the everyday work of many Moscow magi. Depression (likely what Tolia in the example above suffers from) in these terms can be seen as 'semiosis stalled': a painful body-mind state without recourse either to the Object or to the Interpretant. Providing the Representamina for devastating, but nameless and diffuse mind-body states is the mechanism that forms the basis of healing, as studied in the 'meaning-centred tradition' of medical anthropology (for an overview, see Good 1994: 52).

Magic in Russia, indeed, consists to a large degree of generalised psychodynamic treatment, notwithstanding 'changes in energo-information field' that are seen by the practitioners as the main 'locus of efficacy'. The essence of psychoanalysis is precisely the manipulations of subjectivity through management of emotions and passions in interaction between the client and the analyst. It would be interesting to apply the semiotic model of emotions to psychoanalysis, or to compare explicitly the latter and a therapeutic interaction between a magus and a client, but this goes beyond the scope of this study. Rendering the magic treatment in the language of psychoanalysis would be another instance of interpretation, 'professional reduction of subjectivity'. The semiotic model of emotions, on the other hand, might offer a way to approach the subjectivity of the other from a different perspective, from within as it were: through the ways people name their emotions, using one or another term offered by culture (and the ways they switch between the emotion terms available may be significant, as is shown below). Narratives are people's own accounts of their lives; but what happens to narratives in the situations of post-Soviet aphasia (Oushakine 2000), when there is no language to talk about one's experience of transition, liminality and turmoil, private as well as socially shared? This is aggravated by the fact that, as Kharkhordin (1999) argued, the Soviet self, in contrast to the Western subject, is not a 'confessing animal' (Kharkhordin claims that she is, instead, a 'penitent beast' (p. 228), a statement that needs qualification). The Soviet self, according to Kharkhordin, was supposed to be revealed in deeds, whereas the analysis of deep nuances of feelings, characteristic of Western confessions, and, later, of Western psychoanalysis, throughout the Soviet era tended to be considered as useless ruminations and self-digging that belonged to the bourgeois past. Here it should be noted that conversations with friends, especially in the late Soviet period, were characterised exactly by these endless 'self-ruminations'; but this self-analysis can hardly be expected to be found in the stories that informants tell the fieldworking anthropologist. These narratives, however, even if crafted in the culturally specific narrative patterns, are always at first people's own interpretations of their experience. The semiotic model of emotions suggested here can help understand the mechanisms of this interpretation, which can bring us closer to appreciating people's 'social experience', the subjectivity of the subjects who live in a society suffering from 'aphatic paralysis'.

Before looking more closely at the 'logical forms' of emotions involved in particular cases, I want to dwell briefly on the 'grids of power', of which a glimpse is allowed by the episode above. This is well in line with the tradition of 'critical medical anthropology', that has all though its history maintained the focus on medical institutions and therapeutic relations as the loci of power struggle (for an overview, see Good 1994: 57). The relationship between healing and power is one of the main themes of this book, and it will be considered further in more detail with the help of the notion of 'the icon of power'. The power to heal is an instantiation of the more general cultural ontologies of power, and healers' gestalts and their relationships with their patients reflect those 'grids' and 'ontologies' of power discussed in the Introduction. The conversation above, as well, bears clear traces of these grids.

Fundamental to the entire process of interaction between the magus and the client described above is a covert power struggle, in which the client repeatedly tries to take the lead and pursue her own agenda, while the magus shows who is at the wheel. The clients portrayed in this episode present the familiar Russian archetype of the strong mother and her adored son over whom she wishes to exert total control, in the name of a mother's love, and the rifts and wounds it can entail.

Motherly love is a paradigm of love in Russia, the deepest and most lauded of emotions celebrated in all genres of discourse, from the classics to trashy fiction. Motherly love is about as central to emotional life in Russia as is another form of love, its foremost rival and contender – romantic passion between lovers. As in English, these two kinds of love are denoted by the same term, *liubov'*, and in practice if not in normative morality their essence is similar. The totalisation demanded by passion contradicts other commitments; and so the son's beloved may be the worst rival of a loving mother. Grown-up children constitute a valuable resource, not only for the mother herself, but also for the rest of the family. This is evidenced by the vehemence with which Tolia reacts to the mention of his older brother's new woman, the creature who is portrayed as having taken total possession of him, cutting off the pool of emotional and material recourses otherwise available to his cognates. It is striking in this scene how Tolia comes to life when his sister-in-law becomes the subject of the conversation. He would seem to have much at stake in identifying the latter, rather than his former girlfriend, as the perpetrator of *porcha*, and as the sinner liable to receiving hellish punishments.

Tolia's mother is yet one more of those strong women who so abound in Russia. This is a fact that Tatiana does not fail to point out. When she notes that although the mother is also targeted, only the son is affected, she seemingly acknowledges, and pays homage to, the strength of this woman. But she also subtly implies that it is because of this strength, and the resultant imperviousness of the mother's gestalt, that it is the son who must take the thrust of the blow, and bear the brunt of the consequences. Anyone with first-hand knowledge of 'motherly love' in Russia can readily comprehend the struggle between Tolia's mother and his former sweetheart; the girl's frustration when she felt that her fiancé was slipping from her grip, back onto his mother's bosom; and, not least, the girl's mother's disappointment when she realised that her daughter's prospects of founding a family were cast to the four winds.

All these complex emotions, nourished on cultural expectations, norms and realities – the longed-for marriage, romantic love, strong and possessive mothers on both sides – could very well intensify into outright war. They could have likely distilled into blind rage, a bout of sustained hatred that Tolia's former girlfriend and her mother would put into a series of magic activities aimed at harming Tolia's mother, as well as his entire family. Rage is, after all, an alternative to servility and passive acceptance. Rage and hatred that have commuted into magic activity are forms of agency, possibly reinforcing or reviving the person's life force (Kapferer 1997). But the moral origin of these emotions, and of this kind of agency, is highly problematic, in Russia as elsewhere, by virtue of its strong potential for destroying the bonds of sociality.

This is why thwarted love is a most widespread reason for the various forms of love magic – *privorot*, attraction of the loved one, and *otvorot*, repulsion of the rival (literally, turning him away from her; another name for *otvorot* is *ostuda*, cooling off). These operations, connected with manipulating the complex of emotions that comprises what is known by 'love', are usually rendered by magi themselves in normative exegesis as kinds of black magic. Accordingly, the readiness of a magus to undertake such work for clients is considered as a sign of the practitioner's low level of spiritual development. However, castigated and reviled as immoral, the demand for this kind of service never abates. Hence, years on, newspapers are just as full of advertisements about *privorot* and *otvorot* as ever before.

Characteristically magi, as Tatiana here, tend to assume the role of moral tutors. This is nothing new among the Russian health-providers, especially in the areas of health care that are directly connected with passions, such as sexuality and reproductive health. Michele Rivkin-Fish, in her work on post-Soviet gynaecologists and sexual educators (1999), shows how their message tended to depart from health advice proper and to take the tones of admonishment and exposition of moral transgressions (*oblichenie* that, as Kharkhordin [1999] showed, was one of the basic Soviet techniques of fashioning the self). Practising magi are no different in this respect from the doctors in district clinics. However, if the municipal clinics' doctors can be as harsh to their patients as they want, not worrying about losing their clientele, magi, as private service providers, must be more careful not to alienate their paying clients unnecessarily.

But Tatiana does more than just admonish. She attempts to redefine the anger that clearly obsesses Tolia's mother, who has no doubt in her mind as to who the perpetrator is. Hers is a righteous anger (or 'just anger', as Lambek and Solway [2001] put it): she sees herself as being harmed, and craves redress and the punishment of the wrongdoer. But Tatiana appeals to her to curb her anger. She does this admonishing directly, as a priest would do, when she calls on Tolia's mother not to harbour bad feelings against the perpetrator. When one is angry, however, admonitions are of little help. Tatiana knows this perfectly well herself. By urging the mother to adopt the Christian virtues of pity and meekness, and by repeatedly trying to steer her clients away from trying to pinpoint the enemy, the magus points up her status as a preacher and an arbiter of morality. My guess, however, is that she knows full well that her appeals may fall on deaf ears. But she does more: by presenting the semiotic Interpretant of anger as the ultimate punishment, i.e., divine retribution, as a fact, she attempts to halt the semiotic chain of her client's anger, thus removing the disruptive sting of this culturally ambivalent emotion.

If there are some basic emotions that are universal, anger is one of the prime candidates for universality. However, in many cultures expressions of anger are muted, attenuated and transformed, sometimes to the point of being unrecognisable. In terms of the semiotic model of emotions outlined in the Introduction, it is the Object of anger that may be universal: situations where the subject feels unjustly or unduly wronged. The Representamina, the linguistic terms for anger, obviously differ cross-culturally, and may well be absent. The Interpretants, the feelings and actions that ensue when the subject considers herself unduly wronged, may be vastly different, not only cross-culturally, but even within one culture, depending on individual temperaments, dispositions, and modes of upbringing. Lambek and Solway (2001) argue that where cultures offer appropriate mechanisms to process anger, it is prevented from turning into blind rage, and its destructive potential is channelled into socially productive forms. Conversely, Katz (2001) demonstrates what happens when such mechanisms are absent, as in the case of road rage on congested American motorways. To understand the potency of the semiotic operation as effected by Tatiana, I shall now look more closely at the cultural status of the emotion of anger in Russia.

Judging by the amount of violence that has occurred throughout Russian history, and that continues to plague Russian life at every level, the emotion of anger permeates the everyday life of *Rossiiane*. However, the Russian case provides a good illustration of the distinction between anger and blind rage made by Katz and further discussed by Lambek and Solway. What strikes the student of emotions in Russia is that there is no adequate word for the English 'anger' in the Russian language.

There is the word *gnev*, which is best translated as 'wrath'. This emotion is already ambivalent. *Gnevlivost'*, hot-temperedness or a propensity to exhibit strong anger (even if it is justified), is a negative trait in the Russian orthodox aesthetics of behaviour. On the other hand, the expression of *gnev* is acknowledged as being an attribute of Big Men, as in the case of the famous historical figure of Ivan the Terrible, Ivan Groznyi (who, according to the legend, killed his son in extreme *gnev*). The adjective '*groznyi*' is an archaism that means awesome, threatening (from the word *ugrozhat'*, to threaten), or dangerous. It is associated with great and unquestionable power that instils respect and reverence.

Gnev as an emotion term (Repesentamen) is never used in everyday situations (other than perhaps ironically). It is, rather, reserved for literary, ideological and lofty speech, to refer to mass outbursts of anger (or rage), which, while potentially devastating, may well be morally justified. *Pravednyi gnev*, righteous wrath, or *spravedlivyi gnev*, just wrath, is something that the Russian people (*narod*) were said to feel on the eve of revolution, when the burden of abjection and oppression became intolerable. Righteous wrath is likely to be manifest in large-scale social upheavals. Although strong anger leading to actions aimed at retribution and redress, possibly with devastating consequences, is deemed reprehensible by Russian Orthodox morality with reference to the individual, for whom humility, meekness and patience are foremost values, it takes on another hue when attributed to the masses. In that case, it acquires an aura of grandeur that lies beyond human morality.

As there is no exact equivalent to 'anger' in Russian, there is no verb that would directly correspond to 'be angry'. The literal Russian translation, *ia serzhus'*, would not normally be used by people in everyday situations to denote that they are really angry. A mother might say this to a mischievous child, or a lover to the beloved; but, uttered as such, it would always have a tender, forgiving, or perhaps even coquettish nuance. In addition, the neutral statement 'he is angry', rendered by '*on serditsia*', would denote a much milder state of displeasure than the English equivalent.

Even though there is no lexical equivalent for 'anger' in the Russian language, the semiotic Objects of this emotion undoubtedly occur in all human societies, and Russia is certainly no exception. In contrast to other peoples described by anthropologists, who are 'never in anger' (see Briggs 1970), Russians express their anger both frequently and vehemently: talking in an agitated manner, often using *mat*, the famous Russian foul language; threatening each other gesturally, or initiating brawls. Anger is often a central emotion in the emotional complex that drives people to seek the help of a magus, and Tolia's mother is an example of this. Black magic, i.e. magical operations with the expressed aim of harming another person, would be one of the possible Interpretants of the semiotic chain of the emotion of anger in Russia.

This semiotic chain comes to a stop when the angry self is reassured that the situation has been put right. There are many possibilities of terminating this semiotic chain of anger. One is that the guilty party asks for forgiveness; another, that the angry self decides to forgive the wrongdoer, convinced, for example, by the admonitions of others (perhaps a priest), or out of religious piety. Yet another, equally conceivable option of terminating this chain is to ensure that the wrongdoer is duly punished. This is what Tatiana does in her conversation with Tolia's mother, while at the same time relieving the latter of the need to take to redressive action.

Apart from these pragmatic ways of expressing anger, there are, of course, some Russian words that express the emotional state of being angry (the linguistic Representamina of anger). One of them, as discussed above, is 'wrath', *gnev*; another is a uniquely Russian emotion term, that of *obida*. *Obida* can be approximately rendered as the feeling of being unjustly hurt, which results in resentment, irritation, and sadness. *Obida* can be described as anger quenched, directed inward, not given way, where an active expression has been rejected (although there are accepted ways of expressing *obida*, it can perfectly well be denied any expression). In terms of strength of feeling, *obida* is quieter than anger; while anger is active, *obida* is passive.

There are two idiomatic expressions in Russian that involve *obida*, and that hint at the different cultural ways in which the semiotic chain of this emotion can unfold. One is *zatait' obidu*, 'to conceal or harbour *obida*', the other is *proglotit' obidu*, to swallow *obida*. This latent grudge is also referred to in the expression '*ne derzhi obidu*', 'don't bear a grudge [against somebody]'. These expressions imply that the negative feelings of anger, injury and resentment, even if they do not entirely disappear, will not be acted upon. In the first case, that of concealed *obida*, however, their sting, their agentive capacity remains dormant, but retains its potential for triggering further action in future: the chain of signification is suspended, but not terminated. In the latter case, that of 'swallowed' *obida*, retribution or other related action is quenched, and possible redressive action is unlikely ever to come to the surface in social life; for all practical purposes the semiotic chain is terminated.

Tatiana admonishes her client to let go of her anger, suggesting somehow that its redressive work of effecting justice will be brought about by something or someone else. What that agency might be remains unsaid. It may be Tatiana's own magical force, or the Higher Powers that will finally implement this punishment. But the agency of punishment is immaterial. More importantly, Tatiana 'virtualises' the pragmatic Interpretant of her client's anger, absolving her from the urge – stemming from cultural logic as well as from psychological need – to act out its disruptive consequences. While the moral lessons are straightforward, and as all types of sermons may well fall on deaf ears, the changes in the orientation of the self are achieved through the subtle process of manipulation of signs, signs that act on the client's consciousness without the latter being aware of that.

Liuba's redemption

So far, I have tried to show how the magus's role of a moral preacher is augmented by her semiotic manipulations of clients' emotions. While I do not know what happened to Tolia, I had a chance to follow other cases more closely. One of them is the story of Liuba. By the time it was told, Katerina had been treating Liuba for eighteen months, a treatment that Liuba considered an astonishing success. At that time, Liuba was one of Katerina's most devoted clients, and she enthusiastically testified to the transformations which had been wrought in both her personality and her everyday life.

Liuba was a warm and pleasant woman in her late forties, working as an accountant in a restaurant. At the time she told me her story, she considered herself as having recovered, and she was proud of it: she saw this return to life as a feat she had achieved as much by her own effort as by a miracle worked by the magus. She loved and admired her magus. She had accepted Katerina's charisma totally, and she was happy to testify to the magus's power (just as a born-again Christian testifies to the power of the Holy Spirit). Like all those who are saved, and as disciples of charismatic teachers, she was at pains to emphasise the redemptive potential of this power, its greater-than-natural transformative edge. She did this by plotting her story in the canonical way of all tales of salvation, by contrasting the abyss of her despair with the joy of her present life.

Liuba had married young and lived with her husband for about twenty years. She had devoted all her life to him, she did not have any close friends, nor any interests that did not have to do with him. During Soviet times, she was employed at a military factory, and earned good money. It was with her own money that she had bought a splendid three-room condominium (*kooperativnaia kvartira*), an apartment she loved and kept warm and beautiful. She had also bought her husband a car, although she herself did not even have a driver's licence.

In their marriage, he was the moody and unstable one; he never had a job for very long and was continually on the look-out for something. After perestroika, he started to look for ways to make a quick buck, and he often got into trouble. Liuba was the one who represented the family's economic security. When her military factory closed down and its employees were fired, she quickly retrained, and learned accounting. This, and a stroke of luck, allowed her to find herself a well-paid job in a restaurant, a job that enabled her to support her husband while he continued to 'search for himself' as they say in Russia (*iskat' sebia*). She commented on this situation as being unusual, and maybe in a way unfortunate: 'Just at the time when all the women who previously had earned their living were now laid off and were left at the mercy of their husbands, it was he who was a millstone around my neck (*sidel u menia na sheie*). Maybe that was what made him bitter: it is humiliating for a man to be supported by a woman, especially when all his friends are in the opposite situation.' Her husband became restless, and spent lots of time elsewhere, trying, but in vain, to start up some sort of business.

Business in Russia, as Liuba remarked, is not exactly conducive to peace of mind. Possibly because of the nerve it took, but possibly for some other reason, he suddenly became impotent. She took care of him like a mother would have; she took him to hypnologists and psychologists, and was as kind and tender to him as ever, and, gradually, he recovered. She thought herself a happy woman. True, they did not have children, due to some health failure on Liuba's part, and this, initially at least, had caused them much grief. Especially to her, she said, because after all it was her fault. But she thought he had come to terms with that; indeed, it was even better that way, because she could give all her attention to him, to care for him as a mother does for her child. She lived for him, and he accepted it; they *were* a family and that was her most cherished treasure.

Her troubles began when her own mother fell ill, suffered a stroke and became bedridden for six years. Luiba's husband started to spend even more time out, and would come back late, smelling of vodka and neglecting Liuba in more or less demonstrative and humiliating ways. When she tried to reason with him, he became aggressive.

Three years later, Liuba's mother died. 'In a way, it was a blessing for everyone, it spared her further suffering, and it saved me from being the nurse of a bedridden patient, but ... she had been the only person who needed me. And now I felt I was totally alone in the world; I was not needed by anyone (*nikomu ne nuzhna*).'

By that time Liuba's own health was destroyed. She often felt dizzy, would get heart aches and migraines. Her psyche, or 'nerves' as she put it, deteriorated as well. She developed claustrophobia: she was terrified of closed spaces, and she could not stay alone in the apartment, while her husband spent most of his time out. This was when she brought home a puppy, which quickly grew into a huge black dog, a Schaeffer mongrel, 'of rare intelligence and beauty'. With Pirat, she could get through the evenings alone, and she had someone to care for.

Her 'nerves' got worse. She had difficulty sleeping, especially when her husband would come home late, smelling of alcohol, to fall down into bed and start snoring without so much as a word to her. She started to be overcome with suicidal thoughts. This is how she expressed it: 'When I looked out of the window, the trees seemed to be stretching their arms out to me, luring me out, promising to catch me if I jumped. When I stood at a metro station, waiting for a train, the rails would draw me down, like a magnet.'

It became so bad that she was hospitalised in the 'Clinic of Neuroses', a mental clinic that treated milder phobias and depressive conditions, and was less feared and stigmatised than other, more dreaded, regular mental clinics. ('He [the husband] refused to take care of Pirat, of course; a person like him, incapable of taking care of another living being (*zhivoe sushchestvo*). Thank God, my sister took care of Pirat. She was not happy about it, but she realised how much this dog meant to me'.) Her husband did visit her in the clinic, but these were formal visits, no more than five minutes, and he showed no real compassion or affection. When she was finally released, she found her beloved apartment in total disarray: bottles of vodka, heaps of cigarette butts with traces of lipstick. When she challenged her husband, he became violent, screaming. 'What did you expect? Do you want me to end up with a loony?'

Liuba's health continued to go downhill. Doctors diagnosed hypertension and heart failure, and prescribed expensive medicines. She was taking the medicines, but she felt no better for it. One day she fainted, was diagnosed as having suffered a stroke, and hospitalised again. This time, she ended up in a district hospital, in the worst possible conditions. 'Our state hospitals, you can imagine … In these hospitals, if you don't bribe the nurse, you don't even get your bed sheets changed.' And this is how she lay there, alone, on filthy, unwashed sheets. 'People died at night, and corpses were left right there in the corridor for hours, before they took them away. Once I woke up because I could feel an itch in my ear. It turned out that a cockroach had crept into my ear while I was asleep. They had to pour sunflower oil into my ear to wheedle it out …'

When she finally came home, to find it, once again, a pigsty, the husband said to her: 'I wish you were dead'. The real nightmare began. He kept telling her that he wanted her dead; he even told her that he had lit a candle in a church for her to rest in peace (*za upokoi*), a well-known trick of folk black magic. 'He humiliated me, he treated me as if I were not human, worse than you would treat an animal. All the *obida* that I felt … (*tak mne bylo obidno*). Why did he have to hate me so?'

Pirat the dog was the only living being (*zhivoe sushchestvo*) in Liuba's life. 'You can't imagine how Pirat was afraid of him. When he [the husband] came home, Pirat's whole body would tremble, his hind legs would give way, he would creep with his tail between his legs, and pee on the floor. And this was not because he beat him or anything like that. Pirat just knew this man wanted me dead. Pirat

97

was a complete nervous wreck: he would get hysterical when he heard harsh sounds, he would tear at the leash to run away because he was so terrified, and he dragged me all the way after him so that I fell on the earth. He was ashamed of himself, but he couldn't help it: he would panic, terrorised by the slightest sound. My hands were all bruised and bleeding, and I could only walk Pirat at night, when it was quiet in the streets.'

'So, this man wanted me dead. Because he hated me, and because he wanted the apartment. The apartment I had bought with my own money! All my life I had done things to please this man, and now, to please him, I was supposed to die! No, I decided, this was not going to happen! One evening, I called a locksmith [*slesar'*], and he changed the door lock. When my husband came home in the middle of the night, he couldn't open the door. He pounded and hammered at the door, but I did not open. Next day he came with two policemen, to fetch his things.'

'Why should I live any more, I thought to myself. He wanted me out of his life so badly, so I might as well die. One evening, I ran a bath, sat in it and cut my wrists. I started drifting away, and then the pain subsided; I was beginning to fall asleep, when suddenly Pirat started to growl. He growled and growled so terribly, he sat right next to the bathroom door and growled. And suddenly I thought about what would happen to him when they found me dead. They would certainly put him to sleep as well – who would want to take care of this dog, with the state his nerves were in? I thought that I was the only living being for Pirat, and I was responsible for him. So I forced myself to climb out of the bathtub and bandaged my wrists, and went to the fridge and gave him some sausages, the food he likes best.'

'My husband did not turn up, and it was just as well. If he had done at that time, maybe I would have killed him. He wanted me dead, but he would not live to see me dead, and to own my apartment! I did not want to die anymore, now I wanted to live, in order to hurt him. I hated him so much I could not breathe. Sometimes I hated him so much that my eyes would blur over [*v glazakh temno bylo, tak nenavidela*]. I wanted to harm him. They say in the Church that sins should be forgiven, but he never asked for forgiveness. I have taken so much hurt from him, I have been patient with my *obida* for so many years [*stol'ko let ia terpela obidu*], he had hurt me so deeply [*on tak menia obidel*], and now I wanted to hurt him back. I was obsessed by it. I wanted him to crawl back on his bare knees, crushed, hurt, humiliated as I myself was. To punish the bastard!'

'This is when I first saw an ad for a black magus. This was what I needed. I called the number, the secretary answered, I asked her what it would take to punish someone who hurt me (who had inflicted such a terrible *obida* on me – [*kto menia sil'no obidel*] and I started crying. I cried and cried and I couldn't stop. The secretary gave the receiver to the *mag* himself. Stop crying, the *mag* told me, and suddenly I stopped crying. At that moment I believed in him: if this man could make me stop crying, then he could do anything. "Can you really punish him?" I said. "Yes, I can", he answered, "How would you like me to punish him? I can make him die, or I can make him sick, or maybe just impotent? Make an appointment, and we'll talk it through."'

'But I never went to this man. I got frightened, because I felt this man could really do what he had promised. And I realised that I did not want my husband dead, after all ... What I wanted was only that he understood how much he had hurt me, how much *obida* he gave me [*kak on menia obidel*]. That he would ask for forgiveness, that he would tell me that he needed me, that he would remember all I had done to help him ... So, I started to look for other ads. That was when I came to this Centre, to this magus who had put all these flashy ads in the newspapers. She was nice and smiling, but she was totally indifferent ... I told her the story, and I told her I wanted him back, and she said that it was not impossible, but that it would cost me – when she uttered the figure, I almost fainted. I did not have that kind of money. "But if I manage to get all this money together, shall I have him back?" I asked her. "We shall see," she said. "What do you mean, we shall see?" I cried, "I'll spend all my money, I'll get myself to debt, and I might find myself exactly where I stand now?" I never went back to that magus, but I kept looking for other ads, and kept asking around, discreetly. And that was how I found Katerina.'

'I fell in love with her completely the moment I saw her. She was so thin and fragile, she seemed so young and vulnerable, and yet she exuded power. She didn't fawn, she didn't put on false polite smiles, she was as strict and austere as a nun, and yet there was so much love in her. She was the first person in my life who accepted me as I was, who saw me as a human being with dignity, a person worthy of love inside this lame and swollen wreck of a body that I had become by then. I was short-winded, my thyroid gland was swollen, and I cried all the time. I fell into her chair, told her my story and said: "I want him back!" "But why do you need him?" she asked me. "I don't need him! What I need is for him to understand how badly he has hurt me. I need him to creep up to my door, to kick him like a mad dog, to throw him out, so that he would understand what *obida* feels like, for him to be sorry ..."'

"'Let's talk about it later," Katerina said then. "Let's first take care of *you*. Look at yourself! You are reduced to nothingness!"' (This quasi-Sartrian definition of life in a state of total demolition, of the condition on the edge of being human, is a literal translation of a colloquial, and widely used Russian expression *'Da vy zhe nikakaia!'*) "'But how much will it cost? I have only this much money," I said. She gave me a figure, one-fifth of what they charge at these centres, and added: "You can pay me gradually afterwards, when you have money."'

'When she treated me, I don't know what she did, but I felt I was in paradise. I had never felt so good in my entire life. Here she was, sending her energy to me, and she was doing it only for *me*, only to make *me* feel better. It was as if God's love had descended on me, and it was being directed onto me for my own sake. It was for *me* – aging, ugly, swollen, hurt [*obizhennaia*] by the man I have given everything, not needed by anyone [*nikomu ne nuzhnaia*] ... Katerina made me feel as if God still loved me. My *obida*, that had been devouring me from inside, like an ulcer of the soul, simply disappeared. After two séances, my oedema also started to subside. The swelling on my leg had gone down, I stopped limping. I went to Katerina twice a week first, and then once a week. I forgot to take my pills for hypertension, and forgot to go to the medical examination when it was time. I was not afraid of anything, I knew I was protected. As soon as I felt pain somewhere, I took myself off to Katerina, and the pain would disappear.'

'I suddenly felt that it was good to be alive. I had never felt like this before. Just joy, at nothing in particular, simply because I was alive. My husband turned up a couple of times, to pick up the rest of his things. He was apprehensive, but as I did not attack him, we didn't fight, and we parted calmly. I did not want to harm him anymore. All I wanted was to have him out of my life, and I told him so. In fact, what I wanted was to de-register him from my apartment [*vypisat'*], but for this his cooperation was needed, and it was not forthcoming. In the back of my mind I had the thought that he could always come back and claim his part of the apartment, but then I stopped thinking about it. When Katerina was behind me, I knew everything would be all right.'

'The only problem I still had was with Pirat, my dog. He was a total nervous wreck. I still could not walk him in the daytime, because he started at the loud sounds in the street, at spluttering of exhaust pipes, and he would drag me yards after him, through the dirt, so that my knuckles were all bruised and bleeding. The vet prescribed him some tranquilising injections, but they didn't help one tiny bit. Katerina started working with Pirat, too. She gave me a bottle of water charged with some spells that she had read over it. She said it was a spell against fear in people, but that it would work for the dog as well. I wetted Pirat's face with it and gave it to him to drink. Also, she gave me a candle with her spells on it, and told me to light it and draw it in circles around his muzzle and his whole body. Usually Pirat plays with me when I fiddle around him, but when I did these things, he lay as if frozen, totally motionless, his face between his paws, looking straight ahead, as if spellbound. And she gave me this spell against fear; I read it over Pirat, every morning and every time we would go out.'

'Gradually, Pirat was completely free of his fear. I could walk him in daylight, and he was not frightened by noises any more. He is a perfect dog now, these days he never drags me along. And I want him to have a good life. He doesn't eat any odd thing, this dog, I buy meat for him at the market. And he shows me what he wants to eat. He comes up to the fridge, I open it for him, and he points with his nose at what he wants to eat. It's incredible how intelligent he is. Sometimes when I buy sausages for myself, and he wants a sausage, I give it to him and have some tea for supper instead. He is like a child, he does not understand that there is only one sausage left, so what can I do? He is a big dog, and when he is hungry, he feels really hungry, and I can always manage with just tea, it's even better for me if I miss a meal. Maybe like that I'll lose some weight and become a bit more like Katerina.'

'This change in Pirat was a real miracle, but there were other ones as well. I had this old icon, for example, it was totally clad in silver [*oklad*], and I never knew what it was that was painted underneath. And suddenly, one of those days, I looked at this icon and I saw that a small window on the *oklad* had opened, and Our Lady's face was there, her eyes were looking at me! Then I knew I would be all right.'

'As for Katerina, she is now in my life forever. I just love her, that's what it is all about. She never makes me feel bad about myself. She never makes me feel guilty or foolish when I make mistakes. Instead, she always explains to me why I did it, and why I needed this mistake for my development, and what I had to learn, and why I should never do it again. She makes me feel human, always. And God, have I changed? At work, they look at me in a totally different way. Men give me those looks – you know – and they flirt with me! ... I know that I look good now, and I feel young and fit, I run about like a doe on my high heels, I forgot all about the time when I had a limp ... But men – I never let them close. Katerina says that I am not prepared for a man yet, and that when I shall be, we – she and I together – will pull some good man to me, someone to lean against [*podtianem* is a Russian word Katerina uses, meaning to pull or draw, gently but determinedly, as one might tow a boat to a pier by a rope]. But then I think, why do I need a man? If I want to spoil someone, I can spoil Pirat, and otherwise I can take care of myself. I am strong now, I don't need anyone to lean on.'

The conversation with Liuba took place during one of my later visits to Moscow, after Katerina had spent a week with me in Sweden. During this visit, I realised how dependent some of her clients were on her physical presence in Moscow. They called her daily, some even several times a day, and Liuba was among them. One late evening she called Katerna to tell her that there was an emergency. 'I felt so unprotected when Katerina left', she told me in our conversation afterwards, 'that evening suddenly I started bleeding, and it wouldn't stop. I called the ambulance, and they came and gave me an injection, but it still won't stop. They were going to take me to hospital, but I thought about Pirat: who would take care of him when I am away? And I refused. Instead, I called Katerina, and I prayed that I would get hold of her. And I did. She gave me a spell against bleeding, and she was doing some work herself, even though she was in Sweden. And the bleeding stopped. Her power is really extraordinary. But I have also become stronger. *I am* a strong woman, but she helped me to remember that I am one, and she helped me act as one. I am strong, I am responsible for myself, and for Pirat, and I can take the consequences.'

Part of Liuba's treatment process readily lends itself to be recounted in the language of psychoanalysis, for example, of object-relations therapy (as developed, e.g. by Kohut 1977). In these terms, Liuba's affliction can be seen as 'narcissistic disequilibrium', when love of the self is displaced by anxiety and self-hatred. Object-relations theorists posit that healthy narcissism is necessary for an individual in order to forge a connection with the world and to construct a meaningful identity, and this is what Katerina helped Liuba to regain when she challenged her to 'take care of her own self'. This self-love, that, in the West, is assumed to be constitutive of a healthy self, can develop through 'selfobjects', objects of the world which a person can identify with, which she can take inside her self, thus forming a bridge between the inner and the outer world, a 'transitional space' (Winnicott 1958). These 'selfobjects' are formed when the self is mirrored by the other, offering her a moment of narcissistic illusion. Katerina acted precisely as such a 'selfobject' for Liuba, as a therapist sometimes does for a patient in the therapeutic process. As the therapist envisaged by the object-relation school of psychoanalysis, Katerina represented for Liuba 'the grandiose self' or 'the idealized parental imago' (Wolman 1996: 584), that was by Liuba transmuted into a positive self-image. Katerina became for a while a mirroring and idealised selfobject, something in which Liuba could invest emotionally, maybe by way of 'libidinal transference' ('I fell in love with her'): an 'object' experienced as seductive and powerful. In the language of psychoanalysis Liuba's convalescence can be termed 'the revived narcissistic equilibrium' (Wolman 1996: 585), which is experienced as feelings of elation, of aesthetic and moral perfection. As it is also envisaged in psychoanalysis, when the sense of union with Liuba's idealised mirroring selfobject was threatened (by the latter's physical absence), these feelings of omnipotence gave way to helplessness and fear expressed as physical ailments.

Closer to the language adopted in this book, and in an attempt to avoid 'professional transformations of subjectivity' (Kleinman 1995: 96), we can try to discern what the *illusio* was in particular social games Liuba was engaged in. As we can see from Liuba's story, 'what is at stake ... for coherence, for transcendence' (ibid.) is always more than mere day-to-day survival. What is involved in 'coherence' is dictated by cultural definitions of what it means to be a person of worth and dignity. Emotions are always connected with values and are therefore a crucial part of 'what is at stake'. As Kleinman notes, 'to feel is to value or devalue, to connect or to stand apart, to act in resistance or to be paralyzed by our embodied social circumstance and our socially projected bodily experiences' (1995: 177). The transformations of the self that are at the core of healing are predicated on the changes of emotional dispositions and embodied subjectivities, as psychoanalysis also holds. How do we get at these emotional changes, however? Narratives of the self can provide a view on the semiotic complexes of emotions. The Objects are situational configurations that are described by the narrators; the Representamina are names that they give to their emotions (and the absence of names may be significant as well); the actions and reactions (or the lack thereof) are the Interpretants that can vary within the prescribed limits. It is the structures of the semiotic chains, the way people interpret their 'daily rounds of happenings and transactions' (Kleinman ibid.), that might provide access to their social experience, where the individual is 'a bodily nexus of social, relational, moral and political connections', that help discern the stakes in the social games they are involved in.

What was at stake for Liuba, in the beginning of her narrative, was precisely what Kleinman calls 'coherence': her own self-image of a woman of worth. In his study of the Soviet 'background practices' of self-fashioning already mentioned, Kharkhordin (2000) argues for the significance of various groupings (collectives) for the individual's sense of the self. The individual self as it emerges from his study exists insofar as it is included into the network of social relations (p. 195). It is the self that knows itself and comes into existence through, by and for the others. There were those multiple networks, formal working collectives as well as informal diffuse groups of friends that provided the individual with her sense of the self. Liuba's rendering seems to qualify this view. All the networks of others are reduced in her story to only one significant other, her husband. It is through living out the idea of romantic love, of being a good wife, that she has built the self of worth and value. This image, however, seemed to have crushed against the realities of her own practical life as well as those of gender structures. The role of a soft and nourishing wife sits uneasily with that of a strong and independent woman, sole family provider, something that Liuba also seemed to take pride in. This contradiction of gender roles and expectations under socialism has been inbuilt in an uneasy juxtaposition of conflicting gender roles, which Yurchak wrote about (2002). In Soviet times, women were offered contrasting images of femininity. In the public arena the persons of social worth were cast as workers, bosses and party members, while in the private sphere the dominant image of social value was that of a tender and caring woman, mother and wife, the keeper of the hearth. In her study of gender discourses among middle-class men after perestroika, Russian sociologist Elena Meshcherkina (2002) pointed to the conflict rooted in this gender doxa, that was bound to beset both men and women especially when conditions changed. After socialism, when the public symbolism of socialist times completely lost legitimacy, a woman who was successful in her career could become uneasy about her own identity and social role, precisely because she shared gender role expectations with the rest of the society. This was the case with Liuba, who, although proud about her material independence, also saw it as a possible source of the problems that followed.

The roots of the problems people faced could certainly be traced to the past. But it was a general social turmoil, a changed 'background of practices', that finally disrupted the dynamic equilibrium of values, dispositions and possibilities of living up to cultural ideals (even as those ideals themselves were rapidly changing). In her study of the human price of the Chernobyl catastrophe, Petryna (2002) shows how bodily illness and social disintegration lead inexorably to the demise of the self, defined through the bonds with significant others, as much as through the available cultural symbols from which to build the self. The contexts in which the person has come to know herself as an individual of worth and value have ceased to exist; physical, psychic and social death of the individual self and of the 'body social' are aspects of the same phenomenon. In Liuba's case, her social contexts that gave her the sense of self seemed to be of a private rather than of a public or official nature.

This notwithstanding, her individual self is after all defined only through others. She conveys this by the expression 'to be needed by someone', *byt' komu-to nuzhnym*. It is this paramount value that guided her loyalties throughout her story. Thus, the time Liuba had given to her dying mother was taken away from her husband, which she herself saw as the cause of his turning away from her. But what made Liuba choose her mother over her husband was the feeling that she was needed by the former but not by the latter. The discomforts of tending a dying person were for her not only the fulfilment of filial duty; what was primary was the satisfaction of being needed, and therefore Liuba's mother's death was her own social death, also expressed as debilitating bodily ailments. What prevented her from taking her life was, again, the sense of 'being needed', if only by her dog Pirat, the living being who, in her rendering, remained in her life as the only significant other (or 'selfobject').

Her way of caring for her mother, wholeheartedly and with commitment, contrasts in her story with her husband's 'official' visits to her in various hospitals. The horror of public hospitals is a familiar, shared and a richly discursively elaborated emotion in Russia, lavishly evidenced in Russian talk. Liuba's stories of her stay in the hospitals are telling examples of stories heard by any Russian. This horror of public hospitals, undoubtedly founded in everyday pragmatic experience, is also deeply symbolic. It reflects moral and psychological investment in private bonds and modes of care while resenting, disregarding and distrusting the public ones. While in Soviet times the state was a provider of many networks of trust that were quite reliable, the tending of the sick and the old, the care of the body that had lost agency and control, was always reserved for the private relations, primarily conjugal and parental. No matter how strained the relationships between children and parents might be, no matter how much strife marital life brought in its everyday round, the wife was expected to, and would indeed want to, take care of her husband should he become really ill (the converse, from husband to wife, would also be true, though maybe with some reservations). Likewise, the child, especially a daughter, would be expected to take care of her sick parent.

These tacit cultural norms undoubtedly played their role in Liuba's actions, apart from the desire to be needed. If it had been a case of her husband being hospitalised, Liuba's choice would have been much more difficult, and might well have had another outcome. Note also that even the husband, resentful as he was, continued to visit Liuba in the hospital, even if ever so formally. By continuing these formal visits, he kept himself ostensibly within the borders of morality, but he had many ways of signifying that the nature of their relations was anything but amiable marital companionship. Significantly, by choosing to tend her mother, and thus disregarding the needs of her husband, Liuba reasserts herself as a moral person, and the husband's unwillingness to accept this casts him in her narrative as a person whose morality is flawed. It makes Liuba's anger 'just anger' (Lambek and Solway 2001), and likely facilitates the semiological shift in her own definition of the Representamen of her emotion from *obida* to *gnev*. It also morally justifies more active displays of anger on her part. This is the time when her coexistence with her husband ceases to be meek acceptance, an Interpretant corollary of hidden *obida*, and develops into open warfare, a possible Interpretant of *gnev*.

The husband's formal visits, keeping him within the confines of the moral, understandably fail to satisfy Liuba's emotional needs. She feels herself abandoned, not needed by anyone (*nikomu ne nuzhnaia*), left at the mercy of the cruel outside world. The person not needed by anyone is no longer a person at all. His or her social self is corroded, invaded and crushed by the outside world. This demolition of the self, the annihilating capacity of the outside world, is expressed in her narrative by the images of dirt crossing the boundary between the public and the private, a boundary that is meticulously maintained in many everyday contexts in Russia. Thus people are expected to take off their outdoor shoes when they enter an apartment, even if the apartment has not been cleaned for quite a while, and even if it is dry and sunny outside. Housewives assiduously change bedlinen for the family, and people wage incessant and interminable war with cockroaches, the harmless and ineradicable companions of most apartments. These are the widely shared images of the invasion of the outside in the form of dirt (cockroaches are its epitome) into within the self, like the grey, soiled hospital bed sheets coming in contact with the helpless sick body. The most striking of all is the image of a cockroach creeping in through the ear, a primary channel that connects the self to the world, even as it separates the self from the terror and chaos of its noises.

Liuba's story supports the idea first developed by Kapferer (1997), and discussed in the Introduction to this book. In many cultures recourse to the practices of magic and sorcery is a way for human beings to reassert their agency where it has been severely curtailed, and to cement the boundaries of the self where they are fuzzy and permeable. Kapferer, drawing on Sartre, analyses magic as a practice which harnesses human passion, defined as the thrust of intentionality out of the self, towards the field of the Other and the horizons of one's life-world. Passion is a state of consciousness intensely absorbed with something other than the self, be it another human being or an activity within the horizons of the lived-in world.

Like the Singhalese described by Kapferer, Liuba turns to the black magus to restore her agency, to reassert the subjectivity of dignity and control in a state of existential crisis; in a world where to be alone, not to be needed by anyone, is socially and physically deadly. In understanding the transformations of her subjectivity that led to the recourse to magic, it is necessary to dwell further on the lexical Representamina that the Russian language offers for the emotion of anger, that of *obida*. As I have mentioned above, the Object that is involved in the semiotic complex of anger can generate the Representamen of *obida* if one is powerless (while the Representamen *gnev* [wrath] implies that the Interpreter finds herself in a position of power, maybe by force of sheer numbers, as in the case of the people's wrath [*narodnyi gnev*]). *Obida* as a Representamen can also produce different Interpretants. For example, in the case of 'swallowing' *obida* (*proglotit' obidu*) the semiotic chain may be considered terminated, while in the case of concealing *obida* (*zatait' obidu*), the Interpretant is stored in the consciousness of the Interpreter, possibly even acquiring the force of a time-bomb.

There are also cultural traditions and normative prescriptions concerning the moral value of certain semiotic chains, reactions or behaviours. Recall that *gnevlivost'*, an inclination to give way to the expression of one's anger, literally, a tendency to fall into wrath, *gnev*, is one of the vices in the Russian Orthodox tradition. Conversely, meekness (*krotost'*) is a well-known Christian virtue, definitely so in Orthodoxy but also in Christianity in general: the Sermon on the Mount says that only the meek will behold God, and this maxim is made central to Dostoyevsky's moral teachings in, for example, *Crime and Punishment*.

When Liuba turns to the black magus, she abandons the meekness of *obida* and enters the domains of unmitigated wrath ('I hated him so that I wanted to kill him'). In so doing, she recaptures agency, but she steps out of the moral domains prescribed by the Russian Orthodox Church ideology, which extols meekness, condemns pride and anger (*gnevlivost'*) and anathematises all practices of magic. From then on, she does not talk about *obida*, but she conveys that she is taken over by hatred and rage. Both these passions have a semiotic Object of 'anger', similar to that of *obida*. What is different is possible Interpretants. This involves different agentive scaffolding, the stance that the individual (the Interpreter) assumes in relation to the grids of power. The emotion of *obida* presupposes a position of weakness, and is the plight of the powerless; those of hatred and rage (or wrath), and their Interpretants – revenge, retribution and redress- are exercised from a position of power and strength. By reasserting her right to these emotions, Liuba takes the first step in positioning herself as a person of power, a position that she then tries to reinforce by seeking the help of the magi. In this way, she is right when she implies that her redemption is a joint feat belonging both to herself and the magus; it is, of course, none other than she herself who took the first steps.

In her narration of her convalescence, Liuba put the central emphasis on Katerina's seemingly casual remark: 'Let's work with yourself instead.' This appeal to look at one's own self, and to work on 'it', is a commonplace in the West. There, the centrality of 'self', as well as its 'thingness' as a locus of attention, lies at the very core of both professional and pop psychologies, as well as of different techniques of 'working on oneself', 'developing the self', 'taking care of oneself', etc. For Liuba, however, the turn of intentionality towards her self seemed to be a turning point of her entire story. This is easier to understand in view of the main argument of Kharkhordin's study on the Soviet self (1999), already alluded to above: one is endowed with the self only through others, and it is only through others that one can conceive of living one's self as an individual of social worth. Instead of this familiar model, Katerina offers Liuba the self worth attention in its own right, whose source of power and authority lies within rather than without: the model of the self well known to students of Western New Age, but less so to the people who grew up in Soviet Russia. Katerina's repertoire also includes techniques of 'self-affirmation', familiar in the West but less so in Russia: Liuba indicates this when she tells, with some astonishment, how Katerina 'never scolds or criticises' her. The novelty of these therapeutic approaches of 'positive mirroring' is best appreciated against the cultural history of self-fashioning techniques based on the three pillows: 'reveal, admonish, excommunicate'; where the public 'revealing of one's true face' (*oblichenie*) left a person with a choice between conformism and social (and often physical) death (see Kharkhordin, ibid.).

It was this 'positive mirroring' that changed Liuba's subjectivity, which gave her the feeling of tomorrow, the future to project herself into. The subjectivity of rage was replaced by that of hope, which, for Liuba, acquired nearly religious dimensions. This is reflected in the story of the minor miracle: the Russian Orthodox icon painting whose cover suddenly opens up is an index of Liuba's opening horizon, while by its very nature the object itself is both a symbol of Russian Orthodox religiosity, and the icon of the Divine power. The narrative of magical treatment becomes the story of retrieved agency, of redefined emotions, and of intentionality redirected from inside the self to outside, towards tomorrow and the 'horizons of the life-world'.

I would have wished to end this chapter on this note. Unfortunately, the story of Liuba's treatment and her relationship with Katerina had an unhappy ending. Her semiotic chain of anger was terminated, but the structural conditions that underlay the conflict were never resolved; forgiveness of the perpetrator was not envisaged, if only because he never asked for it, and reconciliation never happened. Katerina's treatment seemed to suggest that the further Interpretant of the semiotic chain of Liuba's anger, instead, should be forgetting: 'I want him out of my life'... This is the attitude that many victims take to their perpetrators in other parts of the world. The silent choice to forget, to get on with one's life while banishing the wrongdoer from one's mind, is a pragmatic attitude that can be recognised cross-culturally. These are cultural versions of 'swallowing *obida*' that might work socially, but whose consequences for the individual, as well as the collective psyche, are never finally resolved. Might it be that swallowed *obida* is always a hidden *obida*, a latent threat, a time-bomb?

Liuba wanted her husband out of her life, but practical circumstances rendered it impossible. Liuba and her husband were registered (*propisany*) in the same apartment. This meant that the husband could turn up any time and demand his share of the vital resource, the overall square-metreage of the dwelling area, and this was in fact what happened.

Zhilploshchad', 'living space', is the total of those precious square metres that fuel a multitude of life-and-death battles in Russian everyday life. In Boym's words, 'It would not be exaggeration to say that the major "private" passion in Soviet literature [and, I would add, in Soviet life] … was a passion for dwelling space. … Love, hatred, even melancholy [were] all secondary passions – they usually translate[d] into love of dwelling space [*zhilploshchad'*], hatred of those who have it, and melancholy for lost housing' (1994: 131).

When I talked to Katerina two years later, I asked her about Liuba. Katerina told me, reluctantly, and with utter disappointment, that she and one of her most faithful disciples had recently parted company with bad feelings. One day Liuba had come to Katerina, agitated, her hands trembling, her blood pressure rocketing, her legs swollen. Her main news was that the husband had reappeared on the scene to demand the dwelling space that was due to him. Liuba said that she would rather die. The husband threatened with a lawsuit. Katerina, well versed in legal matters and well connected with legal advisers, tried to calm Liuba down, saying that no judge would ever issue a verdict that could force Liuba to split the apartment if she did not want to. Katerina also offered to find Liuba a good lawyer who would guarantee that she would win a law suit if it came to it. Katerina was even willing to lend her money to pay for this lawyer if Liuba did not have enough.

But Liuba would not listen to any of this. What she wanted from Katerina was to work some black magic on her husband: she wanted him dead, physically out of her life once and for all, and this time she 'meant business'.

Katerina was utterly appalled. She thought that she had worked with Liuba to advance her in her 'spiritual development'. In Katerina's terms it would mean that Liuba should have understood that an evil deed will always rebound on the doer, and that faith in God's goodness and one's own (and the magus's) power will prevail and prevent her from ever again stepping beyond the boundaries of the moral domain. She talked to Liuba rather harshly. 'Whom do you think you have come to? What is it you think you are doing?' It should be noted in parenthesis that now, three years after she had first met

Liuba, Katerina could afford to talk to her clients in a way she could never have afforded before. Her status, her clientele, and the level of complexity of the cases she solves, as she herself puts it, made her much more sure of herself, and much less dependent on individual clients.

While Katerina challenged Liuba, Liuba in her turn challenged Katerina. 'You are not as powerful as I thought you were,' she screamed in Katerina's face. 'You are a fake, and your treatment is a failure! All those years you have been working with me, and look, I'm back to square one.' And so Liuba left Katerina's room, raging, hateful, slamming the door after her. Katerina started to plan how she could help Liuba. She found good lawyers, and new, effective medicines for Liuba's condition of hypertension. But Liuba never came back. 'There are plenty of black magi around, I wouldn't put it past her to give some of them a try,' was Katerina's final, resentful, comment. The power of the magus, ultimately aimed at a moral project of spiritual education and growth, was crushed against the stronger one: the power of material and social structures and the practical attitudes of people that these structures shaped and formed.

Chapter 4
The Icons of Power: Constructing Charisma from the Means at Hand

Icons of power: cultural designs of charisma

For Liuba, whose story is presented in the previous chapter, it took some time to find a person whom she recognised as her personal redeemer. True, she did not give to those she met before Katerina a chance even to try to exert their power over her life; Katerina was the first magus she decided to go for, and she accepted her from the start. In other cases, people do try several magi, part with a lot of money, and experience a number of disappointments before (and if at all) they find the one they think works for them.

In Chapter 1, I discussed the strategies that healers and magi employ to latch on to culturally salient domains of meaning, to present their contested craft as morally and cognitively legitimate. These symbolic domains determine the market sectors of the individual specialists, and allow for the initial recognition that enable two people to meet and to start taking each other seriously. But, if it is to progress any further, healing must involve a certain kind of relationship: the voluntary surrender of one person to another. It involves opening up the boundaries of the self and letting a stranger into the most personal domains, the secret realms of one's love life, family predicaments, business secrets, and one's body underneath the skin. To enable healing, one person has to be willing to put herself into the hands of another, to become the recipient of the other's thrust of intentionality, defined as the power to change. This opening up to healing is akin to transcendence in the experience of being at one with the Divine as described by religious mystics, or to self-transcendence in romantic love, when the boundaries of the self are dissolved and the self merges with the other (recall Liuba's confession regarding the first meeting with Katerina: 'I fell in love with her at once').

Thus, it can be said that healers are taken in by their clients (at least tentatively) as figures of power and charisma, and interactions between them are premised on charismatic bonds. A closer look at healers as charismatic individuals, and at their bonds with their clients, can give a glimpse of a social phenomenology of desire: the emergence of acceptance, admiration and trust that one individual comes to project on another. Elsewhere (Lindquist 2002b) I look at these interactions from the patient's perspective and analyse how they succeed or fail depending on the social compatibility of the parties. Here, instead, my focus will be on healers as icons of power.

In a now classical formulation, Max Weber defined charisma as 'a certain quality of individual personality by virtue of which he is ... treated as endowed with supernatural, superhuman, or at least ... exceptional powers or qualities' (Weber 1964: 329). What makes this interesting in the context of healing, is that these perceived exceptional powers 'decisively shape and reorient dispositions and actions of the followers' (Tambiah 1985: 73). Many researchers after Weber were embarrassed by what they saw as the essentialising and mystifying quality of Weber's definition, the quality that followed logically from Weber's placement of charisma within the individual personality. Scholars after Weber sought to solve this problem by displacing this quality from the individual personality on to the relational dynamics between the charismatic individual and her followers.

Csordas (1997a) developed a basis for further studies of charisma by distinguishing between its locus, its source and its object. The source of charisma, he argued, is based on cultural ontologies; it can be described ethnographically, and it refers to internal orderings and boundaries of a cultural world that defines various conceptions of charisma. The source of charisma can be framed in terms of cultural ontologies of power, and should be analysed as its instance in a given cultural context.

As is often the case with ontologies, those of healing power (and charisma) in contemporary Russia are never verbalised; they are underdetermined, and difficult to elicit. This might be because the power of a healer/magus is of a morally ambiguous and socially ambivalent nature. Not representing any institution, shunned by society's authoritative system of knowledge and morality (science and the Church), magi and healers must draw on these systems illicitly, entering, so to speak, through the back door, into accepted identity spaces.

These ways of constructing the appealing identities that are able to resonate with those of their clients are what I call 'legitimation strategies'. But charisma is something more, something stronger than any legitimation strategy. Charisma projected by the person of power is constructed not haphazardly, but according to certain 'cultural designs' (Handelman 1990). It is a design for penetration, maybe even for violation, whose appeal is strong enough that it opens up the boundaries of the self; but one that is so aesthetically gratifying that it is perceived as salvation instead of violation. This welcome violation of the self, penetration that is invited and encouraged, is due to the workings of desire, and so the models in which the charismatic figures are constructed can be seen as *the cultural designs of the desirable*. Using the sentimental language of popular culture, one can compare these 'cultural designs' with 'keys that unlock hearts'. These keys open up the self and make way for attraction, and for transcendence of the self towards the other.

The locus of charisma, according to Csordas (1997a), must be accounted for in terms of social action and cultural meanings. It lies in the dynamic relationship between the charismatic individual and her followers, and can thus be analysed in its performative and rhetoric aspects. It is a relational concept, which comes into existence only when recognised as such by the recipient (or a group of such, as is the case with the majority of studies of charisma). It is only the recipient's acknowledgement of the power of the charismatic individual that brings charisma into existence in the first place.

Analysis of the dynamics of interpersonal relationships can provide an understanding of how this recognition is granted. Ethnographic details of such dynamics are difficult to provide, because the majority of well-known studies of charismatic power and authority (such as Shils 1968; Eisenstadt 1968; and also Csordas 1997a) study charismatic action of a more classical mode, that between a leader and a quite large group of followers. Thus, most of the ethnographic material pertains to the behavioural and discursive aspects of this interaction, and not to the subjectivity of the individuals in question. In approaching this question of subjectivity, reference should be made to the work of Charles Lindholm (1990, 1995), who likened the charismatic relationship to another sort of passionate interpersonal tie, that of romantic love. According to Lindholm, the comparison between these two modes of relatedness, although so fundamentally different, is possible because both cases include the same mode of phenomenology of the self, namely, that of self-transcendence. Both experiences involve the voluntary opening up of the boundaries of the self, and of the private, jealously guarded life-world. Both result from the choice to let another person in, acknowledging this person's power over the self.

Following this argument, the relationship between a healer and a patient is more homologous with that of romantic love than with that of a crowd and a leader, because it is dyadic, based on immediate face-to-face interaction. Seen in this light, the phenomenological mode of charismatic action can be seen as consummation of the self's desire for the other, the consequence of the self's directed intentionality towards the other, that dispels one's existential loneliness and makes the self malleable by the other, willing to change and capable of change (as, again, is illustrated by Liuba's story).

Seen in this way, romantic love and charismatic acceptance are both forms of desire. But, as feminist scholars discovered a long time ago, 'the head is our most erogenous zone' (see, e.g. Caplan et al. 1993). This is to say that cultural models of the desirable play a part in determining the object of desire, in love as well as in charismatic action that leads to healing. It is these cultural patterns of the desirable that the analysis of the dyadic relationships of charisma can shed light on.

However, there is one major difference between romantic love and charismatic attraction, as Lindholm (1995) was careful to point out. Love (that is, the idealised, although maybe in practice impossible, case of perfectly requited love) is a symmetrical bond between equals, whereas charismatic attraction is profoundly hierarchical, involving asymmetry of power. In contrast to romantic love, in charismatic attraction it is only one of the parties who opens her self up, while the self of the other remains impermeable and closed (in fact, this self-closure is a basic trait of the charismatic individual, as I shall discuss shortly). While reciprocated love is (again, ideally) a perfect balance of give-and-take, of constant openness to the other, the charismatic individual is closed to give-and-take and creates her persona on her own conditions. The charismatic individual is an 'icon of power', and this figure's cultural design must be homologous with those of other icons of power that exist in the culture in question.

The idea of the 'icon of power' resonates with the notion of symbolic types, proposed by Grathoff and developed by Handelman (1991). Grathoff (1970) suggested that in socially dissociative conditions there can appear individuals who are somehow elevated above the context by resynthesising order, by tying together context that has lost its holism. These personalities do so by creating a context of their own, or, more exactly, by becoming themselves a context. They can do so because they are units (in Handelman's words, 'bodies') endowed by their own logic. My qualification here is that this logic is never their own; rather, it is *cultural* logic, the logic of practice and of the accepted cultural order; the logic of the desirable and of the patterns of the 'icons of power' accepted as such in the same cultural system. It is therefore, that the individual can (ideally or temporarily) replace the social order by becoming one herself. It is for this reason that the embodied being of a symbolic type can function as an equivalent of context, albeit on a small scale, as is the case with the majority of Russian healers.

Handelman (1991) suggests that the person becomes a symbolic type when she ceases to be involved in the social negotiations of give-and-take on which every social interaction is built. The insight of symbolic interactionism, that has by now become a commonplace, consists in the recognition that selves are socially constructed through others, through perspectives that combine self and other and are adapted to the reflection of the self in the other. It is this reflection, suggests Handelman, that ceases to exist for the symbolic type. A person becomes a symbolic type when she ceases to modify herself in response to the others, becoming self-referential, a 'totalistic' being or a world onto herself. In the perception of the outside world, such figures can vary from the inhuman (the Madman) to the superhuman (the Prophet or Saviour). The others have only two choices. The first is to reject the vision of reality

117

projected by the symbolic type; the second is to accept the charismatic self as all-encompassing, thereby determining one's own reality in accordance with that of the type. Charismatic individuals are adored by some, hated or ridiculed by others: one man's Saviour is another man's Madman.

For those who accept the charismatic individual as a total being, the world becomes defined accordingly. The followers are ensnared within a self-signifying, self-reifying perspective of the symbolic type. This holism is constructed according to the salient cultural designs of power and desire. This is why the symbolic type can resynthesise disintegrated contexts, turning fragmentation and chaos into a world that is whole, beautiful and desirable.

In this and the next chapter, I shall introduce three practitioners, charismatic individuals whom I met in the field, and whom I came to know sufficiently well to get a glimpse of their own perception of themselves, of their subjectivity as persons of power. All of them enjoyed the reputation of strong healers, all of them had many patients who saw their treatment as successful and who testified to their healing power, to their ability to effect changes in others' lives.

The nun of her own cloister

The first of them, the magus Katerina, has already appeared on these pages. As I have already mentioned, she and I became very close. Subsequently, we shared 'living space' for periods of time, and I had a chance to see her in her everyday life. I witnessed the human and personal cost of a charismatic gift, and I also understood the challenge of meeting such a person face-to-face. It was in this meeting, through its various facets, that she emerged, for me, as an 'icon of power'.

I first made Katerina's acquaintance on the telephone, when I was preparing for my first fieldwork trip to Moscow in 1999. I was studying advertisements for healers and magi, thinking that I should make an appointment with some of them when I arrived. I called several numbers, and everywhere I was asked what kind of problems I had. I had decided from the start that I would not lie and invent a problem I did not have; I determined not to come to a magus as a patient on false pretences. Partly it was the ethical training of the Western anthropologist that required the fieldworker always to be upfront and straightforward, not to conceal one's identity as a researcher nor to pass for someone one was not. Partly, I must admit, I was vaguely guided by the old Russian superstition: if you lie that you have a problem in order to gain a favour, sooner or later the problem will get you.

Therefore, every time my call was answered by asking what my problem was, I tried to say that I did not have any problem, that I was a researcher studying magic. With varying degrees of politeness, the recipients would reply that they did not want to hear about any damned research, and that I should come back when I had real problems. Almost despairing, I came across a small notice advertising, apart from the usual range of services, a seminar for women that promised not to solve their problems for them, but to give them the tools that would enable them to manage their problems on their own. Somehow it struck a more familiar note – Western, feminist and New-Age – in the spirit of 'help to self-help', rather than in the Russian saviour style.

I dialled the number, and a young, sweet voice, clear as a silver bell, answered. I asked about the seminar; it turned out that one course had already been completed, and the other had not yet been scheduled. 'But what are your problems?' she asked me. Anticipating the reaction, I answered that I was a researcher writing a book on magic. 'Very good,' she said, 'I am a researcher myself, I am also writing a book on magic. Come and see me and we'll talk.'

At that time Katerina received patients in the very centre of Moscow, within walking distance of Red Square, in an old mansion tucked away in the labyrinth of tiny side alleys and inner courtyards of the old city. No sign indicated the presence of a magus's consulting room. Instead, there was a nameless door squeezed between the entrances to a computer company and a travel agency. All premises were rented out by a former institute of research and design (*konstrukorskoie biuro*) that had in better times occupied the ground floor of an old, formerly beautiful, but now dilapidated building.

Like many establishments of the same kind, the institute had now lost its state funding and had to make do using every source of income the manager could muster. One of them was to rent the rooms of the institute to the new private enterprises; Katerina's was one of them. The employees of the offices were scurrying about back and forth, with water kettles and paper binders, and were smoking in the worn-out armchairs next to the entrance to Katerina's door. This door carried no clues as to the identity of the business that went on behind it, except for a small paper reproduction of the icon of the Ascension of Our Lady. Sometimes people slipped through this door, trying to avoid eye contact with the other people dashing about the corridors. Clients waiting their turn sat in the waiting room, furnished unobtrusively with two wickerwork armchairs and an oil-lamp (*lampada*) burning under another icon on the wall. The books on the magazine table were about healthy lifestyles and self-fulfilment, of the type one can find in the waiting room of any Western beauty parlour, with the addition of a couple of books popularising the Russian Orthodox religion.

The morning I came to see Katerina was one of those excruciating Moscow mornings at the end of November when it seems that all the elements have joined forces to drive urban dwellers out of their minds. Big wet snowflakes poured from the skies, mixing on the ground with mud and salt, turning into thick slush. Ruts and potholes in the pavement turned into hunting-traps that tried to grip the high-heeled boots and the long coat flaps of Muscovites, ever fashion-conscious despite the hideous weather conditions. The heavy, sticky, cold flakes got stuck on people's faces and in their hair, smearing makeup and turning hairdos into deformed scarecrow-wigs. Zaner (1981) defined effort as a universal existential element that outlines the contours of the self, an insight that Csordas (1997b) developed; but it can also be argued that when effort exceeds a certain limit, the scaffolding of the self starts to creak and crackle. I was in the state of disarray and nervous embarrassment that people feel when losing control over their physical comportment, a state that was bearable only because I shared it with the inhabitants of the thirteen-million-strong city who were unfortunate enough to have to tread its streets that morning.

After a strenuous search through the mazes of old Moscow's streets and courtyards, I tumbled into the room and fell into the chair, totally exhausted. The owner of the establishment was already there to greet me. Being a woman of flesh and blood, she must also have come to this place from somewhere, having to overcome the snowstorm, the rush-hour metro carriages packed far beyond the limits of their capacity, and the slush-covered potholes of the Moscow streets. None of this affected her appearance, however, and in this respect she presented a stark contrast to myself, and to several clients sitting in the waiting room. In the dark room, lit only by a couple of candles and oil-lamps placed on the walls and on the small table between the chairs, she looked very young, maybe in her early twenties, innocent and untouched by life's tribulations. Unlike my own hair, hers was dry and perfectly styled. Her whole appearance was an example of the sublime art of make-up and coiffure that looked so natural that it almost made the beholder forget that this beauty was all man- (or, more exactly, woman)-made. The 'almost' was there to be appreciated by other women, who know what it takes to be beautiful and well-groomed, on a November Monday morning and in a weather like this.

Many Moscow women love to make themselves beautiful and, in doing so, they spare no money on clothes and make-up; these are often the conspicuous signs, or, more exactly, the indexes, of a person's willingness to invest time and money in being attractive. This was not the case with Katerina. In the semi-darkness of her parlour she looked as if she had no make-up at all. Nor did she have any jewellery, not a single ring on her fingers, not the smallest pendant around her neck. Her fingernails were cut very short, and she wore black sneakers and black clothes, long skirt and long sleeves, fitting just tightly enough to outline her small, slim, fragile, but exquisitely built and very feminine body. This austere exterior, so different from the usual attire of Moscow beauties (who love jewellery, perfumes, fine fabrics and tailoring which shows their bodies off to advantage), singled her out as different, above and beyond the more or less widely accepted codes of feminine attractiveness. Her huge, grey eyes stared into yours, unblinking, unsmiling, as if transfixed. She spoke with a pleasant, low silvery voice that was strangely even and flat, as if devoid of emotion.

But most intriguing was her manner of speech. Moscow society is highly stratified, and native sociology is pervasive: people are always keenly aware of their own and others' social position, and can place others almost at first glance. They can certainly locate each other from the first spoken word, as the native sensitivity to speech has always been well developed: people immediately reveal themselves, and place others, by the slightest accent, by subtle shifts of vocabulary and lexicological usage.

With Katerina, all the social markers in her speech were as thoroughly obliterated as those in her outward appearance. As I was to discover later, she had mastered the discourse of all social groups and could talk with everyone in their own language, using the finest nuances of their particular group vernacular: from elite film makers and natural science researchers to small traders from rural areas and ethnic minorities, from old ladies belonging to the intelligentsia to middle-aged politicians and young gangsters (*bandity*).

I told her about my project, and she looked perfectly comprehending and sympathetic. What I needed, we decided, was, first, that she would tell me the basics, how it works, and what the terms mean. We agreed that she would give me lectures, and I would pay her as for a treatment séance; she told me she had given lectures before, even to big audiences. Her lectures, which I taped and transcribed, proved to be very useful; but all my attempts to elicit her personal life story were immediately cut short. From some patchy noncommittal conversations I found out that Katerina was in fact my age, about twenty years older than she looked (in the semi-darkness of her room), and that both she and I had sons in their early twenties. She was a single mother, and spoke with perceptible pride about the beautiful relationship she had with her son; she had divorced his father early on, and she raised her son all by herself.

After further conversations Katerina and I found that we had some other things in common in terms of memories and experiences. This shared background that stemmed from belonging to the same age and social group might have added to an inexplicable chemistry that sometimes appears between people. It made it easier to talk on the personal, human level, woman to woman, and prepare the ground for a friendship that was to develop in years to come. Even so, at this first stage in my fieldwork, it seemed impossible to come close to Katerina as a human being. Perhaps one of the reasons was that, in Russia as elsewhere, human contact grows from common problems and predicaments; for Katerina, it seemed, it was crucial to make it clear that she had none. This struck me as a conscious strategy of self-crafting, and this strategy became clearer the longer we knew each other. She was a symbolic type in the sense that the boundaries of her self seemed to be closed. This came across clearly from the way she handled situations of uncertainty, and their emotional corollaries: anxiety and fear.

In Russia, for every mother with a son in his late teens, one problem overshadows all others: the possibility of military service.

Horror stories about the military abound in Russian talk. Many of those who have experienced serving their conscript term in the former Soviet, as well as post-Soviet, army, confirm that reality is every bit as horrible as the stories. This military service is considered to be especially perilous for boys from the ranks of the urban intelligentsia, since this is a golden opportunity for their contemporaries from other social strata to get their own back on city sissies. To have her boy end up in the army is every middle-class mother's worst nightmare. But there are ways of obtaining a dispensation. There are legal ones – if a boy has serious health problems, or, more preferable, if the boy studies in a college that has a military department in it, which qualifies the students for a dispensation. There are also illegal ways of dodging the draft: for example, paying a bribe in order to obtain a certificate of ill health that would prevent a boy from being conscripted. For people on moderate incomes, usually all their contacts are set in motion in order to collect the required sum of money, and to activate 'connections' in order to make payment possible. For those families whose boys go to the relevant colleges, the important thing is to manage all the strenuous exams, so as to pass to next year's course; if one fails at the exams, one can be expelled and end up in the army anyway. All these are moments of uncertainty that create a good deal of anxiety and fear in families.

In one of our first conversations, Katerina told me that her son was studying in a technical institute, which he did not like because his interests were more in the humanities. He could not choose the education he liked, however, because it did not provide release from the armed forces; and he was hanging precariously between semesters, having failed some of the exams. 'Are you not worried?' I asked her. 'No, I am not', she said. 'I *know* that he won't end up in the army. I just *don't see* him in the army.' She meant her supernatural seeing, seeing in the future, and she presented this ability to see as an explanation for the absence of that fear and anxiety which were part of the life of any other woman in her position.

Once in our conversation I mentioned that the house where I lived in Moscow was fifteen minutes walk from the nearest metro station. I said that I remembered how as a young girl, I was always afraid to walk from the subway, and how my father always used to meet me and walk me home. Now, my father was dead and there was nobody to meet me; I told Katerina how difficult it was, after Sweden, to re-socialise into the feeling of fear that permeated the air in Moscow, including the fear of walking the streets after dark; how this constant fear drained me. I asked her if she was afraid to walk to her place from the subway. 'Of course not', she said very firmly, 'Nothing bad can ever happen to a magus!' On another occasion, we were discussing the horrors of the public health care system, and I asked her whether she was not afraid to fall ill. 'A magus cannot fall ill', was her answer.

Over the years, as we became friends and I gained insight into Katerina's personal life, I had many opportunities of witnessing how she managed its inevitable blows. Several times she was evicted from the premises she worked in. Having no place to work was catastrophic for her: not only was she the single breadwinner for herself and her son, but she was paying an astronomic price for her son's college. Her failure to pay could mean his being expelled and subsequently conscripted to the army. In spite of what she said about a magus never falling ill, her own health turned out to be precarious; several times she had had to be taken to hospital by ambulance. The enormous concentration that her work required only aggravated this condition; but she could afford no respite in her work, not even lightening her load a little, because she had to pay for her son's education. At one point, when she was evicted for the third time in two years, she decided that she had to save money to buy herself and her son an apartment of her own. This pressed her to work even more. No sooner had she got together the necessary sum of money than she had something like a stroke and had to be hospitalised. Her hospital stay devoured all the money that she had saved, and when she was released from hospital she had to start over again from scratch.

In short, Katerina's life was as full of uncertainty, danger and helplessness as that of millions of her compatriots at that time. Like them, she had every reason to experience the fear and anxiety that ensue when agency is severely retrenched, when life is out of control, when help can only be hoped for but never counted on, much less expected or demanded. But, there was never a hint of strain in her voice, never any concern on her brow, never any agitation in her manner. Asked how her life was, she had a standard answer. She used to say: 'A magus's life can be just fine or very fine. With me now, everything is very fine.' Only a couple of times was life 'just fine': when she was diagnosed with a disease that was chronic and required long and expensive treatment; when all her savings were gone after her stay in hospital; when her son failed a couple of exams and was in danger of being expelled. As comment, she always said: 'Nothing bad can happen to a magus. This is just a karmic knot that I have to unravel, that is why it is given to me now.'

And indeed, her problems were always solved one way or another. There were grateful clients who helped her find a new apartment to live and work in when she was thrown out of the old one; and every new place was better than the old. When she lost her savings, a rich client gave her money as a gift; yet others would lend her money on interest-free, indefinite loans. She had a network of informal contacts that reached into every corner of the Moscow world, from doctors and lawyers to politicians and parliament members, businessmen, tour agents, policemen, estate agents, sauna attendants, and more. These were the people that she could activate when she needed them, and that she used with mastery to help her clients in practical ways even as she treated them through the use of magic. She found job opportunities for the unemployed, contacts for those who needed to hire tutors for their children or to pay a bribe for entrance exams into prestigious colleges (usually tutors from the same college are also the conduits for the bribe, even if they do not take the money themselves but only indicate the right people to pay). Katerina found medical specialists and rare medicines for specific diseases, and referred people to car mechanics when their car needed repairs; she connected apartment dealers with those who wanted to sell, and sent out-of-work builders to those in need of apartment renovation. And she used these networks in the cases when she herself was in trouble; people who had no obligation to her but whom she hoped would nevertheless be there to help when she needed it.

This type of contact net, which provides Russian people with no security but which gives them hope of survival in every situation, has been in Soviet times, and still to a degree is, the basis of life for many Russian urbanites. This form of 'barter based on personal relationships, to acquire goods and services in short supply' (Ledeneva 1998: 34) is generally known as '*blat*' (although this word was almost never used by the people who were involved in this type of networking, especially not in relation to themselves, a part of the strategies of 'misrecognition', that, as Ledeneva showed, was an essential part of this system's functioning). The phenomenon of *blat* and its post-Soviet transformations were discussed exhaustively by sociologist Alena Ledeneva in her influential *Russia's Economy of Favors*. In Soviet times, this network of connections constituted essential social capital for people, when it supplemented the networks of entitlements that people had by virtue of their belonging to hierarchies of social power: workplaces or party membership. In a way, networks of blat were structurally homologous to those of magic: they represented alternative channels of agency, used by people to augment their power or to carve out alternative power structures for themselves in the system where it was unequally distributed.

Ledeneva stresses the importance of affective components in the connections of *blat*: it was embedded in intimate relations, and defined in terms of friendship and mutual help, help that could prove crucial in conditions of scarcity. Her discussion of gender aspects of *blat* (p. 120) indicates that *blat*, as well as magic, could be considered as a tool for 'empowerment' for those whose structural conditions in the society made them additionally vulnerable: women were more involved in *blat* than men, and single or divorced women more than married ones. Parallels between magic and *blat* are also hinted at in Ledeneva's quotations of critical descriptions of *blat* provided, for example, by the Soviet satirical press (goods and services are described as materialising 'by magic', in situations where they were unthinkable to obtain by officially accepted means). Her description of a woman who acted as a node in multiple networks of these connections, a doctor by the name of Natalia, also, in some aspects, reminds me of Katerina. (Natalia is referred by Ledeneva as *blatmeister*, a word that was all but an outright insult in Moscow in my times, and so I would be reluctant to apply it to Katerina, even if the essence is much the same). Ledeneva compares this type of activity with that of brokers in network analysis, with their role as intermediaries between different social circles. By virtue of their liminal social position, they could use their contacts as resources, but were not members of any one of them, just as the case was with Katerina. Another similarity is a talent, a special psychological make-up that this position calls for. As Ledeneva's informant expressed it, 'people felt that I had weight ... I was told many times that I talk well ... It was a confident tone that made people do things for me'(p. 109). It should be remembered that

Natalia was a hero of Soviet times, while Katerina acted in the post-Soviet period, when the ideas of power and the structure of its icons had undergone considerable changes. Among the most important transformations of informal networks, Ledeneva notes the fact of increasing separation between instrumental and affective components of human ties. It should be noted, however, that this separation is never absolute or final. As before, people in Russia tend to seek 'personalization of bureaucratic or other formal relations' (p. 83), or, as an informant to Dale Pesmen (2000) put it, 'Everybody wants something, but only through somebody.' Also, Ledeneva is correct in pointing out that blat is still crucial when it comes to information exchange, distribution of lucrative jobs, and getting services of better quality for those who are not rich enough to buy it all for money. Katerina's clients, and Katerina herself, belong to precisely this category, and so it is understandable why Katerina's informal networks were both part of her power as a magus (her charisma) and indispensable for her own survival.

These safety nets, maintained by socially competent people in both Soviet and post-Soviet times, can be compared with those officially provided by Western welfare states: in both cases, they help people survive when all else fails. There is, however, one crucial difference between Katerina's safety networks, and those provided by Western welfare states. In the latter case, people are *entitled* to some modicum of social support; for Katerina and her compatriots, this is not a matter of entitlement, but, rather, a matter of hope. While networks of *blat* are in many cases about improvements in lifestyle, in some cases they are a matter of survival, as when it comes to getting access to better health care, or acquiring dispensation from the military service for one's son. Moreover, even though in the post-Soviet environment much of what was before provided by *blat* is now bought by money, money itself is an insecure resource: it can be plentiful today but gone tomorrow, or its owner could be there to enjoy it one moment, but dead the next, killed by a hired gun. (This is reflected in the profile of ailments among Katerina's clientele of rich male businessmen, who come to get relief from anxieties, phobias and severe depressions.) If hope is one aspect of uncertainty, coupled as it is with desire, fear is its opposite, dark side: fear can be seen as the desire to avoid painful consequences (Kulick: personal communication). Being two sides of desire, hope and fear are both connected with uncertainty; they both arise when agency is in question, and when the boundaries of the self and the contours of the life-world are under threat.

When Katerina talked about her life, she never displayed fear, nor did she express hope: she did not *hope* for the best, she *knew* that it would come. '*Nothing bad can ever happen to a magus*'; Katerina's predicaments were, in her rendering, not misfortunes to decry but lessons to learn, so many welcome opportunities to unravel more karma knots. She constructed her persona in markedly neutral terms with regard to the signs of fashion, luxury and social distinction; and she tried to ensure that the boundaries of her self were impenetrable to external impulses. In her work with others, she said, she 'opened up their channels'; in contrast, she *was* in the channel herself. As part of her treatment, she routinely sent people to church, to light a candle, and to pray to God. She herself talked to God, but she never prayed in the sense of humble supplication. When she worked with a client she created out of her or him a human being that was always improved as compared to the one that first came to her, as a desperate human being in a shambles. As she lived her own life she was continually creating a totally perfected human being out of her own self. As she once let slip in conversation, to be able to work, she had to talk to God; but when she was working, she *was* God.

This statement of the divine mission may sound like an expression of utter hubris, a sin of pride (*gordynia*) much derided by the Russian Orthodox Church. It also appears to chime poorly with the highly mundane nature of Katerina's assistance to her clients. This paradox, however, becomes more understandable in view of Max Weber's discussion of 'active asceticism', an ideal-type category that he defines as 'a god-willed *action* of the devout who are God's tools', and which he contrasts to 'the contemplative *possession* of the holy, as found in mysticism' (Weber 1970 [1946]: 325, emphasis in original). Active asceticism, according to Weber, operates within the world and seeks to master it. This mastery includes the world's 'natural' aspect, the needs of the body, which means to 'tame what is creatural and wicked through work in a worldly "vocation"' (ibid.: 326). This is very much in line with how Katerina disciplines her body, abstaining as much as possible from 'the needs of flesh'. But this mastery also includes the world's 'sociocultural' aspect, which means to be able to navigate its structures pragmatically, armed with a sharp, sober and calculating mind. Indeed, as Weber writes, in Katerina's gestalt asceticism is 'rationally active': it shows 'its Janus face': on the one hand, abnegation of the world, and on the other, its rational command (ibid.).

Talking about Katerina as compared to an ideal-type Weberian charismatic, another aspect of her attitude must be mentioned – her attitude to money. As I have shown, the trade of magi is a professional occupation, which allows some women (as well as men) to find their economic niche in the disintegrated economy. In the previous chapters we have seen how aptly some magi make their clients part with their money (recall the encounter between Misha and magus Zinaida in the Centaur centre). Katerina charges her clients as well, and her everyday survival, as well as her more far-reaching dreams of enlightenment, depend on her clients' financial support. But we have also seen, in the example with Liuba, that Katerina refrains from wrenching people's arms, from squeezing out of them as much money as possible. Indeed, sometimes she does treat people free of charge (and sometimes people do tend to take advantage of that, trying to go for a free ride, somewhat to her consternation). In this ambivalent attitude to money, Katerina seems to correspond, once again, to Max Weber's theories of ideal-type charisma. Even though Weber as well admits that 'even a pirate genius may exercise a charismatic domination, and charismatic political heroes seek booty, and, above all, gold' (ibid.: 247), he sees charisma, primarily, as based on rejecting 'all economic conduct, ... any pecuniary gain that is methodical and rational'. This is the main feature that, for Weber, distinguishes charismatic authority from bureaucratic and patriarchal authority. Just like the great sociologist, who elaborated his ideal types being well aware of their lack of correspondence to the real world, Katerina attempts to be an ideal type in her own ideology and self-presentation, while constantly negotiating her survival in the real world.

When we first met in her parlour on the ground floor of the old house in the centre of Moscow, she was a good informant. She shared with me her esoteric knowledge without reservation, she was calm and focused, and she had a surprisingly good grasp of the research I was doing. There was no way, however, to get beyond her impermeable public persona, to get insight into her life behind the façade of the invincible magus. She bluntly refused to recount her 'life story', to tell me how she became a magus and what she did before. After three lectures we exhausted the theory of magic as she conceived it; I wanted to hear more about specific cases, but her sense was that this was more of a subject for leisure-time talk, and leisure time she did not have, nor did she want to spend it with me. I wanted to see how she worked with clients, but she said that my presence at the séances would embarrass them unnecessarily. Some friends of mine asked me to take them to Katerina, and I agreed on the condition that they would allow me to be present. After the first conversation, Katerina told me that they were behaving unnaturally, that I was making them shy, and that it was unfair to make their treatment more difficult with my presence. Some of the acquaintances I commissioned remained her faithful clients for a lengthy period; but when I came back a year later and wanted to talk to them about it, they refused to discuss it, saying that it was 'just psychotherapy'.

At the end of my first stay, I invited Katerina to visit me in Sweden, and she agreed. When she came and stayed for a week, our relationship was redefined, from that between a researcher-client and the ritual expert-magus, from between anthropologist and informant, to that between two friends. Katerina described for me some cases in detail; and, with much reluctance, she gradually started to talk about herself.

Grudgingly, and in broad but meagre strokes, she painted me the picture of her life. In contrast to Liuba's narrative, which although outwardly so dispassionate, had been so passionate in essence, Katerina made a strong point about passions being follies, finite and ultimately forgettable. Unlike Liuba, she did not want to present herself as unfairly hurt or wronged – exposed to *obida*; her spent passions were welcome lessons, necessary steps on the road to becoming a magus, an icon of power.

Katerina's story

Katerina had grown up in a family belonging to the so-called 'technical intelligentsia' – a social grouping somewhere in the middle of the Soviet hierarchy of social prestige and material well-being. Her father had been an engineer, and the family had moved around frequently. As a girl, Katerina never felt that she belonged anywhere. When she grew up, she also got an engineering degree, and later obtained a job at a factory. There she was moderately successful; she did well professionally, she had, in her words, a 'man's mind', so technology was not a problem for her; but the work did not engage her. With the start of perestroika, the factory was closed down. Unlike many of her female compatriots, Katerina had no problem finding a new job: she was good at figures, and gained employment as a financial manager in a successful and growing private company. She had a good, disciplined mind, a strong *'mentál'* as she put it, and she was greatly appreciated at her workplace.

This was a time when esoteric teachings started to flood Moscow, and 'the paranormal' became an everyday subject of conversation. Charismatic healers treated thousands of enchanted spectators, who filled stadiums and sat glued to television screens. Spiritual teachers from India as well as transpersonal therapists and Reiki healers from the USA and Europe came to Moscow to lecture and teach courses. Katerina soaked up the new philosophy like a sponge, devouring the reprints of Nikolai Rcrikh's works, as well as the translations of Alice Bailey and Carlos Castaneda. At the same time, she discovered that she was good at stage-acting, and she joined an amateur theatre group where she starred in several productions.

She had her son very early, and then divorced her husband, painlessly. He was a good man, but she did not love him. Later, she fell in love with her second husband, and that was *that kind of love*, the love of her life. Her husband was a creative person, a spiritual seeker, an artist, a poet and music-maker. Katerina was good at singing and at playing the guitar. They gave concerts together, singing his songs; they also went to lectures and together discovered esoteric wisdom and the sciences of astrology and numerology. All the while she supported him by working as an economist, while he made music and sought spiritual enlightenment. They had a comfortable life, and she was happy, until one day her husband told her that he was passionately in love with another woman. He did not want a divorce, he wanted her to understand that he was an artist and had to succumb to his passion, while she was his life-companion. She told him to leave.

In her narrative, Katerina neither expounded on her emotions nor castigated her husband. The way she characterised her inner state was that she was 'mortified', 'dead inside', 'annihilated' (*nikakaia*). This was how she found her way to a magic parlour (*salon magii*), a big flashy one, featuring one of the best-known names in Moscow. It cost money, but she earned well, and money was no problem for her. Like many clients of magi, she first sought out a magus to mend her broken heart. But she was proud. She did not ask the magus to bring her husband back. She did not want him back; she wanted him out of her heart, out of her life.

The magus agreed to treat her, and it worked: after a period of treatment, she no longer felt any pain. Moreover, she stayed at the *salon magii*: she realised that she could work herself. Her love was gone, but her 'channel' was open. Her healer became her mentor; he taught her simple skills, and he allowed her to receive clients. She discovered that she was efficient: her clients perceived that her treatment worked. She left the security of her well-paid job as a financial manager and started to work for the magic parlour. After a year she came into conflict with her boss and former mentor – she did not go into detail – but her reputation was already sufficiently good to open her own practice. By the time I met her she had been working professionally for about three years. At that time she used to advertise, but she soon stopped doing so: clients came to her by recommendation, her reputation spread by word of mouth.

During the three years that I have known her as a friend, Katerina has been extremely consistent in her ways of being, in her strategies of self-presentation. She is a strict vegetarian, and she eats extremely little. When I first met her, she ate once every two days; after her stroke and hospitalisation, and after a bout of fainting, diagnosed as blood-vessel problems, she changed her eating habits, and she now eats once a day, a small handful of cooked vegetables and a tiny piece of bread. She is an excellent cook, and she cooks good-quality food for her son, who is also a vegetarian. A sausage never defiles their fridge, but Katerina can enjoy a meal of fish in a fine restaurant. She claims that she has conquered one of the most basic needs of the body, the feeling of hunger. She eats not because she is forced to by hunger, but to give her body some very minimal and basic nourishment. On rare occasions she can break her own rules, joining a family meal or deciding to eat a cake in an elegant café, for company's sake; not following her own canons slavishly, but not exceeding the limits she has set herself for her own indulgence (she would still never eat meat in any form).

The style of her clothes and make-up is still austere, although she pays close attention to both aspects. She always works only in black, and she never wears jewellery; but when at leisure, she wears lighter colours, carefully chosen to match her light grey eyes. Her sight is not good, but she does not own a pair of glasses, using always and only contact lenses: 'a magus in glasses is a joke'. Her clothes always fit tight, to emphasise her slim body in an exquisite petite format. She exercises when time and her state of health permit; her latest favourite is roller-blade skating. She looks young, almost unnaturally so for her age, and takes pride in it: she likes to think that she can challenge, if not entirely bypass, the laws of nature. She can be sprightly and attractive if she chooses; she does not smile often, but when she does, it is a playful and mischievous, child-like smile, so surprising on her visage that one is taken aback.

Thus, Katerina comes closest to Weber's ideal-type charismatic, an active ascetic who lives in and off this world, 'to tame what is creatural and wicked through work in a worldly "vocation"'. The world around her seems uncontrollable, from the hazards of formal structures and informal sociality, to the frailties of the ailing and ageing body. Katerina struggles with all these elements of chaos through a two-fold strategy: first, pragmatically, using her charisma and social competence to activate alternative social and cultural channels of power and agency; and, second, emotionally, by wilfully closing the boundaries of her self to the influences (she calls them energies) that she deems 'bad': those of vexation, fear, disappointment, despair: all the emotions that stem from frustrated desire. Not confined by any authorities or institutions, she is her own authority and an institution in herself. To live up to her task of self-perfection, it is important that there be no failures in her activity as a magus. Any such failure would be a crack on the surface of this icon of power, and therefore, she has to redefine failures as successes, at least from her own point of view. As long as her clients accept her definitions, they remain her clients; otherwise, they leave. But as long as they see her as she sees herself, they are open to her charisma: to her power to change their lives and their selves.

The limits of the charismatic bond

I define my relationship with Katerina by the term 'friendship', a notion that is heavily charged in Russia. Digressions on the semantics of this term appear elsewhere in this book, and I shall not dwell on it here. I shall only remark, referring, for example, to Crick (1992), that it is always somewhat problematic for an anthropologist to designate her main informant as a friend. The relationship between a researcher and her informant is always that of mutual utilisation, not to say exploitation. Katerina was for me a priceless source of information, as well as a doorway into the field. For her part, she certainly enjoyed coming to Sweden and taking a break from her monastic life of dedicated service to the development of humanity, work that was often psychologically frustrating and physically excruciating for her. Still, in a way our relationship was unique also for Katerina, as far as I understand. Early on I realised how lonely she was, a feeling that she later confirmed, in a matter-of-fact way, without either sadness or complaint. (She felt herself as lonely as God the Creator must be lonely where He is, she once noted.) Men were afraid of her, she said: they wanted her power to solve their problems, but they were not willing to offer consistent support in her daily life. They were ready to stand up and to offer practical help in crisis situations, such as finding a new apartment or a place in a decent hospital, lending money or a hand in moving houses, but they were unable to share her inner life (Katerina always hastened to add in the same breath that she did not need it anyway). Her clients, pleased with what they perceived as positive changes in their lives resulting from her treatment, could invite her to a restaurant or to a theatre, or offer her a vacation at a luxury spa, gestures that she always accepted with an easy grace. But, as she told me, they always disappeared when bigger commitments were involved.

This was the case with Gennadii, a successful businessman in his early thirties. Although it yielded good money, his business was never secure: competitors were fierce, money necessary to maintain turnover was often difficult to come by, clients delayed payment for orders, and he could never rely on his partners. All this was part of a businessman's life, and he was coping with it himself; this was not the reason why he turned to Katerina. Still, in the course of their work together, he used to follow her advice in his professional as well as private life, and his business thrived as never before.

Gennadii's main complaint had to do with health problems. He suffered badly from insomnia and agoraphobia: when he had to climb out of his car and find himself in a public place, surrounded by strangers, he was gripped by an uncontrollable panic. He was taking tranquillisers, but they were interfering with his potency, and he started to have difficulty concentrating. After several séances with Katerina, his symptoms disappeared, and his life picked up in all respects. He was a faithful patient and a grateful friend to Katerina for more than a year, helping her out in practical situations. Like several of Katerina's rich clients, he promised her that when a really big deal came through, bringing him a large sum of money, he would invest in her life's dream.

That dream was a centre of her own, where she could run courses, train students, give lectures and seminars: a place of enlightenment in line with her project of 'development of humanity'. Like others before him, however, Gennadii forgot these promises when he got back on his feet. When a big business deal went through, and he did not turn up to say thank you, Katerina understood that the treatment was over. He disappeared from her life, which she interpreted as a sign of her own success: he was so well that he did not need her magical protection any more.

Relationships between a magus and a client that resemble friendship (dispensing mutual help through thick and thin, as well as spending quality leisure time together) are terminated when the client feels that the magus cannot give her or him any more. As Katerina remarked several times, when people get their power back, they think it is theirs, and they do not want to think back to the time when they first came to her, annihilated or 'reduced to nothingness' (*nikakie*). During the three years I knew Katerina, I witnessed several such rich clients who remained on the scene for a while, lending her a generous helping hand, but who later invariably disappeared.

If, deep down, Katerina was perfectly justified in feeling bitter (feeling *obida*), she never let this emotion slip in any of our conversations. She always chose to see severances of bonds as proof of her success, the complete fulfilment of her mission: once these people got from her what they wanted, they could progress further and start living their lives for once, even if they gave up the idea of 'inner development'.

In describing Katerina, a magus whom many of her clients consider powerful, I have tried to show how she constructs her gestalt as an icon of power, or in Handelman's terms, as a 'symbolic type': largely and consciously on her own terms (or so it would seem). The boundaries of her self are, as it were, semi-permeable: on one level, her interactions with people are organised not as give-and-take but rather as her giving and others taking what she gives. This is reflected in the way she envisages the emotional dynamics of her life; she tries to hold her self impermeable from external impulses, from other intentionalities. She has excluded from her life two major forces that, for ordinary people, violate the boundaries of the self and achieve self-transcendence. This is true for self-expansion as explosion, as in love, as well as for self-annihilation as implosion, as in fear. The price she pays is loneliness in human terms, but the power to change others by plying her trade.

This cultural design is strong enough to open up other selves, to make them accept her in her role, and this is the basis of her efficacy as a magus. But the nuts and bolts of this efficacy lie on another plane as well, that of everyday pragmatics. In real life, especially in Russia, people can only function as competent social beings through an endless chain of give-and-takes, through the incessant social exchange on the micro level. Katerina's vast networks, her strong '*mentál*', and her keen knowledge of Russian life, make up another element of her efficacy.

Chapter 5
Charisma of the Office: Healing Power and Biomedical Legitimacy

In the previous chapter I described a lone magus, a nun in a monastery of her own making. In Weberian terms, hers is 'charismatic legitimacy', constructed without reference to anything outside her own self. Katerina has shunned institutional settings as frameworks for meaning or as sources of legitimacy; she has placed herself above and beyond any of them, be it Church, science, bureaucratic structures dispensing conventional biomedicine, or the new structures of business like the Centaur centre. The price she pays is exceptional loneliness and exposure to the manifold dangers of Russian life.

Other healers choose different ways. In the example of Tatiana from Centaur, I discussed the costs and benefits of belonging to an institution, with its social moorings and internal hierarchies. Apart from practical questions of greater security, connection with such institutions can account for a different kind of charisma, the Weberian 'charisma of the office'. It has been argued that charisma is imputed not only to individuals, but also to institutions, symbols and material objects. This has to do with their presumed connections with the culturally envisaged sources of fundamental power or vital force (Geertz 1977; Shils 1968). Accordingly, charismatic individuals may construct themselves using symbolic means that, through their cultural conventions or habits of interpretation, can act as icons and indexes of power. They are constituted as such not primarily by dint of their personal qualities, but, rather, by the person's perceived connections with the sources of established social authority. Obvious examples are the Pope or the President of United States, whose 'charisma of the office' is so strong that the 'personal charisma' of the specific office holders becomes less relevant. Geertz calls this 'tapping into symbolic, discursive and performative resources offered by the culture, implicitly referring to the entities bearing ultimate, order-determining power' (1977: 151). Since these symbols of power are different for different social groups, but also shared within a cultural ecumen (and maybe even cross-culturally), the number of followers must depend on the breadth of the symbolic base on which the charismatic individual draws to create her image.

In this chapter, I shall describe the practitioners who, like Tatiana, chose to identify with the powerful social institution of biomedical science. However, this identification is never complete, since it is never fully reciprocated: just as the Church will never bless magi, its de facto missionaries, so biomedicine never goes the full way of accepting healers into its fold. Therefore, charisma of the office is not enough for a person to successfully ply a healer's trade; individual charisma must also be in place. In this chapter I shall show how healers construct themselves as icons of power, employing various patterns of the desirable recognisable from the Russian cultural repertoire. A cultural psychologist would have invoked the notion of archetypes, but I find this term misleading: it implies too high a degree of both stereotypisation and conscious moulding to do justice to the uniqueness of the people I met. I am also conscious that tracing their traits to the familiar cultural icons can smack of social reductionism: any schemes of interpretation can hardly account for the vital force of their gift, tangible to some, denied by others, and always precarious as it exists only intersubjectively and transiently, as long as it is confirmed by its recipients. Healers, human icons of power, are in Russia prophets for a day: to keep on earning their living by their gift, they must resort to all means at hand to construct and reconstruct their charisma every day anew. It is in the fine fabric of their lives that the clues to their charisma may be found. Therefore, I let the description of this chapter speak for itself, to let its protagonists recreate themselves as icons of power in the myriad of minute details of their daily grind: in their professional and business transactions, in performances of outward beauty and sexuality, and in presenting their life stories, whose value for me lies less in their factual content than in their capacities for performing the narrators' social persona.

In describing the quasi-medical establishment that is the site of this chapter, I also have a broader ethnographic goal: to give a glimpse of the field of medical care in post-Communist Russia. While there is a vast area of medical anthropology dealing with multiple medical care in the Third World, very little is written on the subject for the post-Communist countries. This chapter approaches the field of Russian medical care through the back door, so to speak: clinics like the one described here are a kind of bastard of the conventional medical care. Still, people who work there invest significant efforts in being accepted as a part of it, both by biomedical authorities, and by the users who pick and choose in search of therapeutic efficacy. By looking closely into the everyday world of a healing clinic, we can start forming an idea of what the bigger field of biomedical care looks like.

Nina and Georgii were at the time of my fieldwork working in the same establishment. They were old-time buddies, colleagues dependent on each other, fighting against the tough outside world, as well as rivals covertly fighting with each other for limited resources. It is through these struggles that they cast themselves as figures of [healing] power, framing their charismatic gift of healing, the gift that was acknowledged as such by those around them. This gift was felt by themselves and experienced by others as bodily sensations, and it had even been repeatedly confirmed 'scientifically', in laboratory experiments. However, in itself this gift was far from sufficient to ensure a smooth and trouble-free life for them. It is this continuous struggle for recognition of their power to heal, and their personal project of crafting themselves as the icons of power, that was the focus of their lives, and that will be the focus of this chapter.

The empress and her empire: the Nina-S centre

The site described in this chapter was called 'Nina-S', an abbreviation for 'Nina i Sem'ia' – Nina and her family. Originally, this centre was conceived by Nina as a family enterprise, where she would work together with her two sons, who, she told me, also had strong healing abilities. Both of them had chosen other paths: at the time of my fieldwork one was a surgeon in a major hospital, the other worked in a private garage as a car mechanic. Although somewhat disappointed, Nina understood her sons' choices: they had families to support, and, by exercising their chosen occupations, both of them earned much more money than Nina ever did through her centre.

Nina was a striking woman in her early fifties, a woman of force and stature. She was beautiful and attractive: this she was well aware of, was unabashed in flaunting it, and cultivated it by all means available. Her hair was cut very short, in a bold, latest-fashion style, and dyed flaming red. Her make-up was rich, bright and conspicuous at all times of the day, irrespective of her mood and physical disposition. Her clothes were decorative, intricate, in bright colours and with complicated designs, works of art meant to arrest the gaze. In addition, she wore high-heeled lace-up boots, replete with press-studs.

She made no bones about being a beautiful woman, and she cultivated it using all the tricks of the art. She emphasised her staggering figure by low-cut tight-fitting blouses and jewellery. Her skirts with slits exposed her beautiful long legs with full round knees. Hers was the beauty of a mature woman, at the peak of her powers, self-assured in all her roles and modes of behaviour. Her style of socialising was open, amiable and inviting. She gave of herself freely and was generous with the time and attention she lavished on everyone who crossed her path. She also had an explosive temper, and when she considered it appropriate she would speak her mind in tones of voice that made people shiver. In short, she was the familiar type of the Russian Queen Mother, adored, admired and emulated but also feared when in wrath. She was a matriarch, a self-willed autocrat, a hot-tempered but kind *Matushka* (a diminutive of 'mother', bearing connotations of endearment and tenderness, an affectionate name in Russia for an abbess, for the local landlady of a rural estate, and also the name by which favourites used to address their tsarinas).

I was introduced to Nina by a fellow ethnographer, who had worked with her earlier and could vouch for her healing gift. Nina met me benevolently, and accepted me without hesitation. In contrast to Katerina, who was extremely reticent about herself, Nina willingly narrated to me her long and eventful life. She cast herself as transparent; she had nothing to conceal; she was all there, straightforward and up-front, to love her or leave her.

In the beginning, she treated me as a guest from the media, a familiar figure inasmuch as both Nina and her centre had appeared in the media before. She was keen to show me around, and to present her establishment in the best light. Later, however, she forgot that I was a guest doing research, and accepted my presence as one of the many at the Empress's court. She loved to talk to me when she had a respite from her many tasks and challenges; she read through her archives of medical records, she did not mind being taped; and she shared with me the difficulties of her past and present life. She treated me as she did the rest of the people surrounding her: as a mother treats her children, with indulgence and generosity.

The only thing she could not help me with was talking to the patients. At that time – in 1999 – the centre was at its lowest ebb, the consequences of the financial crash of 1998 still being painfully felt. Nina had planned her centre for 'the usual people', and only a year before it had been quite affordable for the middle class; now, there were precious few who could afford to pay even the moderate prices the centre was charging.

In 1999, when I spent some weeks at the centre, it occupied large, albeit somewhat dilapidated premises on the ground floor of a huge Stalinist apartment-house: a spacious, pompous, and relatively prestigious residential building. The staff consisted of two healers (Nina was one of them), two masseurs (one of them was also a specialist in ultrasound diagnostics), two secretaries who answered the phone twelve hours a day, a bookkeeper, and a logistics nurse.

The latter, Tania, though technically speaking not related, was very central to Nina's 'family', and contributed to the distinct family feeling that the centre projected. She was Nina's best friend and right hand. She took care of many minor practical details, always seeing to it that staff working with patients would have newly laundered and starched white gowns, an essential feature in terms of maintaining the resemblance to a medical clinic, and important for the self-definition of the centre as an institution within the biomedical health-care system. It was Tania who always made the tea that people drank incessantly, that was offered to guests and visitors whenever they popped in, and that counterbalanced the formal clinic-like air of the centre, lending it the welcoming atmosphere of a family kitchen. It was Tania who always kept Nina company when the latter wanted to discuss a new problem with the business or a new item of clothing.

'Nina-S' was a licensed healing centre that advertised itself as treating biomedical conditions. Its official name was 'Health and Treatment Centre' (*Lechebno-ozdorovitel'nyi tsentr*), and with it went a licence number, proudly displayed in advertisements as well as on the billboard that was mounted at strategic places on the outside of the house. The ads, the billboards and leaflets available at the centre also offered the list of diseases the centre promised to heal: it contained, by and large, all possible ailments of inner and outer organs from top to toe (the usual range of diseases that healing centres of this kind promise to cure; see Chapter 1).

Usually, cancer is one of the very few diseases that is not included in this list. It is believed to be too dangerous for the healer, gravely ruining her own energy field and eventually maybe even causing cancer in herself. In this case, Nina was an exception: she was one of the very few healers that I know of who was not afraid of treating cancer. Actually, she had had several patients diagnosed as having cancer, including children; and she told me that all of them were alive and well after working with her. They would come back regularly for preventive treatment, and otherwise felt fine, she told me.

To be able to advertise as a biomedical clinic, the centre had not only to obtain a licence, but also to renew it every year. One of the requirements for obtaining such a licence was that all the healers on the staff have their own private licence, which they could obtain only if they were in possession of a degree from a medical college and a certificate from one of the so-called institutes of traditional medicine. But this was not enough: the centre had to be inspected by official state health-care organisations each year. This was a terrible ordeal for Nina the Director, and required both thorough paperwork and keen social competence in dealing with the intricacies of Russian bureaucracy, both its formal parts and its informal interpersonal relations. The effectiveness of healing had to be judged by the same yardstick as that of biomedical healing – objectively, scientifically, that is, on the results of conventional tests. Every patient who applied to the centre was asked to bring with her the results of all the required tests: blood and urine tests, X-ray pictures of spine, bones and internal organs, ultrasound images of tumours of ovary and prostate, or constricted kidneys. After the first and the second course of treatment at the centre, the patients were sent back to the clinic, to undergo the above types of tests once again. For that, the medical records that the incoming patients delivered to Nina were carefully stamped by the secretary when the patient paid for each successive séance of treatment. These records were kept by Nina in a special cabinet, readily available to the health authorities should they want to take a closer look at them. Much to Nina's frustration, nobody cared to study these cases, the objective testimony to the efficacy of her treatment. But the presence of these case records, completed on special standard forms borrowed from biomedical clinics, was a requirement if the license of the centre was to be renewed. According to Nina, there were some cases when the medical authorities did take the records away for inspection, but they never commented on them, and neither did they ever send them back.

Therefore, Nina invested heavily in equipment that could demonstrate 'objectively' and 'scientifically' that positive changes had indeed occurred and that the treatment had been efficient. One of them was the ultrasound machine, which confirmed the disappearance of myomas, intestinal polyps, or kidney stones. Another was an electrocardiography apparatus that registered improvements in the heart. The object of Nina's special pride was the AMSAD apparatus for computer diagnostics.

The apparatus for computer diagnostics, a ubiquitous feature of medical as well as magical centres, is a device that deserves detailed description in the light of the earlier discussion on iconicity. Its design is based on the idea – also inherent in bone-setting and its many ramifications, and in different schools of 'manual therapy' (analogous to Western chiropractic) – that all diseases of internal organs are conditioned by disturbances and displacements of the vertebra of the spinal column. All viscera are said to generate subtle electromagnetic currents, different depending on the degree of disorders in these organs, which are registered on the palms of the hands and on the forehead. The patient, in the first step of diagnostics, is given two shaft-like electrodes, one to hold in her hand and the other placed as a band over her forehead. The program is then said to measure these currents and to translate them graphically onto the computer screen. By the magic of computer programming (whose mechanisms are totally opaque to the program users working in these clinics), the screen displays the picture of the spine, with all its vertebra in different colours, and a schematic picture of the inner organs, also in different colours and connected by straight lines to the vertebra with which they are supposed to correspond. The legend on the same picture deciphers the colours: from light yellow to dark violet and black, through shades of green, orange, red and blue. The light colours correspond to good conditions, the dark to the various stages of disease. In this presentation, the patient instantly can see the inside of her body, its condition in terms of the gravity of disease, the diagnosis that biomedically is supposed to correspond to her symptoms. The pictures on the screen are conceived as icons of the physical condition of disease, the supposed disturbances in the patient's body. At the same time, these pictures are indexical signs, generated by complex physical mechanisms at work in the patient's body, mediated by computer technology.

Nina (and other healers in other centres, including those of the Centaur type) insisted that patients take these pictures before and after treatment with them. Once, in a mood of exasperation, Nina explained this to me in the following way: 'People are nasty. When they are here, they rise from the couch all elated, saying that they feel so much better, that their pain has disappeared and that they are full of strength. But once out in the street, and back at home with their families, they say that they don't feel anything anymore, that they threw away their money for nothing. It's different when they see with their own eyes how their viscera and vertebra change colour. Then they *know* it worked, not only *feel* it.'

All those iconic confirmations of improvement might well be meaningful for the patients, as Nina suggested; I never became closely acquainted with any of them at the Centre. It was obvious, however, that for Nina herself, as well as for her colleague Georgii, these indicators were at best secondary. Clearly, Nina and Georgii received their most important feedback not through machines, but rather through the patients' own assurances. If the patient did not come back, they were left in doubt: was it because he or she was cured and did not need treatment any more? Or was it because the patient did not feel any improvement at all and went on to seek other treatment? Or was it maybe because she didn't have enough money to come back?

This doubt was never spelled out: like Katerina, Nina could not afford to doubt in her own power, even if others dared to cast doubt upon it. Nor did she ever question her colleague Georgii's healing abilities, even if she was critical of other aspects of his behaviour. The patients who returned to the healers with words of gratitude and admiration were enormously important for both of them: they provided the only definitive confirmation that their healing really worked. In line with the intersubjectivity of charisma, their power existed only when acknowledged and accepted by patients, and it could endure only in their recipients' feedback. At the time of my fieldwork, especially for Nina, there were not many people who could provide such returns, possibly because the relationships between her and her patients were not cast as personal relationships between a charismatic leader and her followers, as was the case with Katerina and, to some extent, with Georgii. They were rather constructed as anonymous and contingent encounters between the humble sufferers and the bureaucratic biomedical machine. All the more valuable were the people who did call back with praise and acknowledgements of improvement.

Both Nina and Georgii presented themselves as primarily biomedical doctors within the confines of conventional Western medicine. This identity demanded that they should cooperate with other researchers in their study of the paranormal. As I mentioned before, these studies had been done in secret under the supervision of the KGB during Soviet times (or at least rumours had it so). This research 'came out of the closet' and was intensified after perestroika. Both Nina and Georgii had in their time taken part in some of these experiments. Georgii, for example, told me that he could overexpose photographic paper hidden in a closed envelope, and change the pH of a chemical solution: feats that he mentioned in passing and dispassionately. It was clear that he did not give much weight to them; he was only being cooperative, helping science along.

Nina had also previously taken part in scientific experiments. Unlike Georgii, she retold them for me several times, with considerable pleasure and pride. In one of them, Nina was given two sets of Petri dishes where cancer cell cultures were grown. Her task was to kill the cells in one dish, and to boost them in the other; and also to heal or to develop tumours in infected experimental rats. She was fully successful with the first set of tasks, while she failed completely with the second. In the first Petri dish all the cancer cells died; and, while the infected rats never developed tumours, the cancer cells she was supposed to boost did not grow better; in fact, their growth was also somewhat inhibited.

These experiments were obviously important for Nina, for they carried symbolic meaning beyond the evident indexical signification of her healing power. This was the only time in my work with healers that the failure to achieve a task was recounted with such enthusiasm. And no wonder: in addition, these experiments constructed her as a moral person. They defined her gift as designed to fight evil, not to assist it, even if for experimental purposes, in the name of science.

According to the rules of the Ministry of Health, the laboratory control of the results of the healers' treatment was formally required for the renewal of the centre's licence. Such monitoring was welcomed by the healers themselves, because it confirmed their power to cure indexically, and because it symbolically placed them within the official health-care system. Much to their disappointment, this monitoring was in fact nonexistent: even on the rare occasions when the district biomedical clinic did collect the case records, it never got back to Nina with any comments. Her explanation was that they were overburdened, which was certainly true; however, it could be also read as a symbolic rejection. Nina was painfully aware of this and spoke bitterly about the arrogance of the biomedical establishment that she had to face throughout her life. This did not, however, make her allegiance to it waver in any way.

There were many other requirements in order to renew the licence. There was sanitary control, when a special representative of the state sanitary inspectorate came and checked if 'sanitary-hygienic standards' were being complied with. There was an inspector from the social security department who checked the bookkeeping to see whether tax and staff premiums were being properly deducted from revenue. There was fire inspection, which checked that the premises were not a fire hazard. In today's Russia, with its complicated bureaucracy inherited from Soviet times, there are thousands of rules and regulations covering all the minutest details. However, the documents in which these regulations are recorded are not readily available to the administration of the centres, and may well be absent altogether. Therefore, the inspectors, the individual representatives of different authorities, who are theoretically in the know concerning these rules, and who are in possession of the stamps conferring the legal status on the certificate, have unlimited power over all sorts of small entrepreneurs (see Lindquist 2000b).

The bribes, the pension funds, the rents, the laundry, the advertisement and the rest devoured all the money that came from the patients. Even in better days running a clinic had not been a lucrative enterprise, but now Nina was hopelessly in debt. She was considering closing the centre and receiving patients privately in her apartment. This was not so easy, however, because she did not own one: she lived in a small, rented, one-room apartment together with her husband, also a non-Muscovite. Also, she felt responsible for her staff, who, as she said, were like a family to her; without her, they would all be out in the cold with no means of subsistence.

Licensing was far from the only ordeal that Nina had to endure as the director of her centre. There were many others. The owner of the premises would harass Nina from time to time, demanding a rise in the rent. In new colloquial Russian these attacks are called *'naezzhat''* and deserve special explication, inasmuch as they are an everyday aspect of any businessperson's life and fight for survival. Literally, the word *'naezzhat''* is used to describe a vehicle running over and crushing a human being. In everyday colloquial metaphorical usage, it denotes an encounter with a superior raw force that confronts the weaker one suddenly and aggressively, without prior notice, with inordinate demands and under threat of violence. An example of *naezd* (the substantive of the verb *naezzhat'*) is when the 'roof' (*krysha*), that is, a gang of bandits who exercise informal protection of a business against other bandits, start demanding of their protégés higher prices for their services. Another example is a visitation of a landlord on a tenant. A rent might have been the subject of prior agreement and due payment by the tenant, when out of the blue the landlord demands that the tenant pay more or leave (or just asks her to move out, without any reason, as happened several times to Katerina).

In most cases, the tenant has no means of protecting herself and has to give in. For a practising magus, it entails a dramatic cessation, possibly even full termination of her activities, because her clients lose touch and might not be able to locate her again. The only way for the magus to cope with this is to place a new advertisement, an expensive business. Nina trembles with rage with she talks about her landlord. So far, she had managed to control the situation, because her husband, young Valerii, himself a professional wrestler, has friends with fists: he used to work for the famous OMON (OMON is an abbreviation for the special-purpose troops that are within the Ministry of the Interior. They are used to deal with internal riots and are staffed with the toughest men around and reinforced with the most modern and efficient equipment). Nina forcefully brings this fact home to the landlord, in her own words, responding to his demands by saying 'You, son of a bitch, just try to do something, and they [Valerii's friends] will smash you to pieces.' So far, this strategy of threatened retaliation has worked well, and the spacious premises have remained at her disposal for a couple of years.

Lack of clients was ruinous for Nina, and at the time of my fieldwork the centre was kept going owing to the help of Nina's husband, Valerii. He was in the lucrative business of delivering oil to the 'near abroad', the neighbouring former USSR satellite countries, and he could afford to help Nina out – the gesture of a real man, as she said. At the time of my fieldwork, however, his business had suddenly come to a halt: the company delivered a train-load of oil to Belarus, but the recipients had refused to pay. Valerii was in the process of negotiating with his OMON friends, but in the meantime his own landlord had closed down his office for non-payment, and he and his companions had turned Nina's consulting room into their temporary office. While one or two patients lay on Nina's couches, her hands doing their healing job over their bodies, three men sat around in the same room, at Nina's desk, talking on the telephone, smoking, drinking tea and exchanging the odd remark with one another. The situation was dire: the negotiations with OMON friends seemed to come to a standstill because Valerii and his companions had no money for the required advance.

Money had to be obtained elsewhere, urgently. Nina started milking her connections; she contacted a former patient, a female customs officer who ran a storehouse of confiscated goods. These goods come in imported batches, but if the import dues are for some reason not paid by the consignees, the goods are seized and become the property of the customs. The director of the storehouse then sells the goods in bigger or smaller batches to interested sub-contractors. The price of a batch is incomparable to the sum demanded by the OMON avengers, but with luck it may be sold off to make up the required sum. For that, the initial sum must be procured, but this is the next question, Nina says. She is displeased with Valerii; he does not spin fast enough, she feels, and she is tired of her consulting room being turned into an office for his business. If Valerii does not start to spin really fast, she says in frustration, she will kick them out of her room, and probably she will even kick Valerii 'out of her life'. For the time being, Nina's consulting room is combined with the men's business office, and none of those involved seems to be too uncomfortable about it.

It is a delight to watch Nina at work. The patient lies on the couch, two huge candles burning behind her head: flame draws out bad energies, explains Nina. She chats on the telephone, holding it deftly between her ear and shoulder; she briefs her daughter-in-law about her grandson's success at school; she admonishes Valerii or any of his business companions present in the room; she gives Tania practical instructions about the laundry; she lectures me about the tribulations of the healer's life in Moscow; or, she talks to the patient lying on the couch, in a warm and motherly way, listening to his or her private problems. All the while, her hands live a life of their own. They are like independent beings with their own agency, seemingly in no contact with the owner, in no connection with what she is at; beings with their own power of expression, aesthetics and style of movements. These movements are confident, generous and sparing at the same time, now fluttering around the whole body, from head to feet, now resting on the sick parts of the body for longer moments. For the inflamed tissues, the movements are soothing, quenching, as if she is extinguishing tiny loci of burning flame, putting out sparks or smouldering charcoals with her palms and fingers. With other types of inflammation, the movements are smoothing, levelling, as if she is ironing out the surface irregularities of an actual tissue. With kidney stones, she moves her fingers drawn together in a pinch very closely to the surface of the body, as if dissolving the foreign tissues with the heat her fingers emanate (this is also her verbal description of what she does). Sometimes she grips and draws out, or rips off, as in the case of polyps or small cysts; sometimes she stirs or mixes the energy of the bio-field, so that it is evenly distributed all over the body, in the way one would stir salt to dissolve it in water or mix the water in a bathtub to ensure an equal temperature all over.

Nina seemed to accept the independent agency of her hands, their iconic and indexical mediation of some higher order of power and knowledge, when she repeatedly assured me that it was her hands that 'knew' what to do, and that 'they' have known it all along, right from the start and throughout her entire life, when she did not even dream of becoming a healer. Nina's self-construction, which could be discerned from her life-narrative, was marked by this never articulated, but perceptible, tension: between being a part of something greater – the folk-village tradition, the scientific medical system, the family – and being all by herself, sprung from nowhere, standing alone and strong, giving to all, but taking from no one. It was a tension between the assertion of individual agency as the source for ordering the life-world of the self and others, and the denial of this agency in favour of being mediator of a greater power, be it of a divine 'higher force' or that of reason and science framed by the biomedical establishment.

Nina's story

Nina was born in a small town in middle Russia. These were difficult times, soon after the war. Her father died when she was a child, leaving the family in a half-ruined house. Her mother raised her three daughters alone. It was a peasant household, and all four women took part in tending the vegetable patch and looking after the cow and pigs that gave them food to survive the starvation of the postwar years. To earn more money for her daughters, the mother had several menial jobs: cleaning, acting as a night watchman in schools, taking in laundry for other people. In Nina's words:

'Our mother was famed for her temper, and she brought us up very severely [*v strogosti*]. We were afraid of her anger [Nina used the word *gnev*], and she sometimes treated us with a stick, but I am grateful to her: she taught us hard work and iron discipline. And she was at the same time both just and kind. She had strong healing abilities, but we never spoke about that subject, we pretended it did not exist: this was a taboo then, and she wanted us to grow up as modern women, not full of village superstitions. But she was known in the neighbourhood and beyond, people would come to her with their problems: "Stepanovna, my newly-born cries all the time! ... My cow has no milk!" My mother would whisper over the baby or the cow, and everything came right again. She never accepted money for her help, but people would bring her eggs and honey, or vegetables from their allotments. But she never taught me any of her arts. It was not like what these other people say: my mother never passed on her secret traditional knowledge to me, holding my hand when she was dying.

Why should I lie and say that I have inherited the knowledge of healing? I have inherited nothing! I am just myself. [*Ia sama po sebe*]'.

'In fact, when I was a child, I would never do anything of that when she was around; she would get very angry with me. She worked hard to give us education, so that we should have a better life then she did. But even when I was a small child, people would come to me with their pains. When I was in my late teens, I had this reputation in the neighbourhood: as soon as someone fell and hurt himself, they would come running to me, I would hold my hand on their scratches, and they would disappear. My mother stopped scolding me for doing that, and started to ask me to cure her head- and back aches, as well. But this was just a part of our life, nobody ever called me a healer, we never discussed it. On the contrary, I used to be a little cross with people when they came to me for healing; I would say: "Do you think I'm some kind of a clown or something? If your head aches, here's an axe, cut it off!" We would laugh about it, but my hands would be doing their job, and people's aches improved … At that time I did not give it a thought.'

Nina graduated from a Teachers' College, moved to a larger town, and started to work at a police office, taking care of juvenile delinquents. There too, her colleagues and her clients used to ask her to lay her hands on the aching parts of their body to sooth their pain. And she loved to work with people, she told me, to help these young people solve their problems, and find the power to clamber out of the quagmire they had got themselves into. At that time, she was married to her first husband, and was already a mother of three.

Nina was working with young criminals, her older son was studying to enter a Medical College, and Nina was studying with him, to be able to help. This was how she developed a passion for medicine. While her son became a full-time medical student, she took correspondence courses at the same college, in a town in middle Russia, and duly got her MD degree. She understood that this was her life's calling. She loved to work with patients, and patients adored her – especially old people, she told me, because she talked to them as much as they wanted, she came to their homes and helped with practical chores, she drank tea with them and listened to their problems. With all her patients, she not only listened to their heart and lungs with the stethoscope and prescribed medications; she also laid hands on the ailing parts of their body, and they felt better.

She was happy, this was what she wanted to do; but her assistant nurse declared war on her, and on her healing methods. 'This was because these nurses like power, they want to be the boss in the doctor's consulting room, to decide how the patients should come and go. But with me, she could not be the boss, my time was scheduled for the patients only, they could even come after hours and chat. She started to report on me: she told my superiors in the polyclinic that I was practising some kind of sorcery. They warned me several times, they said it was a modern scientific clinic, not a place for village quacks [*mrakobesy*] and then they told me that if I don't stop, they would fire me and sue me.'

'I stopped healing, and then I fell very sick. I would faint several times a day, I could not sleep because of nightmares, and when I was awake, I was in pain all the time. Doctors could not say what it was, and I was just withering away. They told my husband to take me away: they said I needed a change of climate. The children were grown up by then, and so we left. We got a contract far away, in Northern Siberia, in a little mining town; you could get there only by helicopter. I got a job there as a doctor. I had a small clinic all to myself, a hospital, a consulting room, a rehabilitation ward, a gym – they were very well-off from extracting metal ore. At first, I tried honestly to work as an ordinary doctor. Once, soon after my arrival, I went to the mine director's office, a big tough guy, and he was sitting there, his head between his knees, writhing in pain. He was having a stomach ulcer attack, he had called the helicopter to be taken to the hospital in the nearest town, but there was a snow-storm and the helicopter had been delayed. "Let me help you. Come to my consulting room," I said. He grumbled that I was talking rubbish, but he was in such pain that he came down and lay on the couch. This was the first time I saw his disease, his ulcer, and again, I didn't know what my hands were doing, they were just doing their job. A half an hour later, his pain disappeared. He kept coming back, twice a day for five days until the storm calmed down. And when the doctors finally came to take him to the hospital, he refused to go: he said he was fine. "I don't know how she did it," he said, "She did some magic with her hands, that's all." They took him to the hospital for tests, colonoscopy, ultrasound – the ulcer was gone! There was not even a scar!'

In a small town like this, the mine director was an almighty emperor, and Nina became his favourite. Rumour about her spread far and wide, and a veritable pilgrimage started. She would receive up to sixty people a day, running a whole hospital with two wards, and using her healing energy to the full. This was the happiest time of her life, she told me, when she saw that her healing worked, and that she was really needed by people (*nuzhna liudiam*).

A year passed like that, and then the powerful healer lost her ground at exactly the point where other Russian women of power usually do: she fell in love. Nina left her husband, and he moved away from the mine settlement. This perfect love lasted for five years: a period of great happiness that ended in hellish pain. Her beloved was torn between his passion for Nina and his family of a wife and two small children, and eventually he made his choice. 'I don't blame him', Nina said, 'He was a noble spirit, and he did the right thing. I was never angry with him. But that was the only time when what they call "paranormal abilities" opened up in me. How I hated it! He was thousands of kilometres away, with his family, and I was as if immured in the wall of his apartment, and this wall was as if made of glass, and I saw everything that was going on, day and night. When he called me, I would tell him: "In that situation, this was not the best way to behave … And then, you called her my name, why do you do this to her, she doesn't deserve it …" All I said was correct, and it was horrible; the worst thing was that I could not get rid of it, I was not in control any more … I had to leave that place.'

The time was late 1980s, perestroika had begun, and a wave of interest in the occult swept over Russia. What had been a suspect and semi-underground practice could now be legitimised in various ways. The healing gift was no longer a silly village superstition, but, instead, the sacred ancient tradition of the occult as well as the science of the future. Nina realised she was not alone with her strange gift, and that she could practise her art without being regarded as a village dummy or a weirdo. She came to Moscow to try her luck. After months of hardships and the precarious existence of a provincial newcomer in the magnetic and monstrous metropolis, she ended up in one of the Institutes of Traditional and Folk Medicine.

It was at that time, the beginning of the 1990s, that a spate of healers, all referring to 'tradition', flooded the Moscow market. 'The Bishops of White and Black Magic' rubbed shoulders with the 'Best shamans of Chukotka' and with 'the White Tibetan Lamas', and competed with the 'Authentic Village Russian Orthodox Babushkas' and the 'Magisters of Cosmology' on the pages of the numerous advertisement newspapers. The medical and academic establishment tried in vain to bring this unruly medley under control, by demanding, among other things, the licences discussed above. Private schools, academies and courses that awarded Professors and Academics diplomas mushroomed, claiming to be equal to the degrees conferred by the conventional academic institutions (that previously had commanded considerable prestige on the Moscow scene and saw themselves devalued by them). Several Advanced Courses of Folk Medicine represented attempts to professionalise healing as an official occupation, and to endow it with a semblance of bureaucratic legitimacy. They did it to achieve a degree of standardisation of treatment, by formulating a theoretical paradigm that could encompass different varieties of healing; by imposing some kind of testing of the healers' abilities; as well as by putting the healers through a standard training course. One of the best-known of such institutions was the centre of Traditional and Folk Medicine, started by Galperin, a psychologist with a solid academic background, faith in healing, and sprightly entrepreneurial talents.

The entrance exam for this Institute training course has already been mentioned in the story of Tatiana in Chapter 1. The gist of it consisted in that a healer faced a patient, a person she had never seen before, and was asked to make a diagnosis. Nina had already had the experience of using her inner X-ray vision before; she told me that she always saw all the ailments of her patients as if their body were transparent. As she recounted this, she noted in passing: 'This, of course, is a totally different level of mastery compared with what I have now. Today, I don't waste my powers on diagnostics: there is medically approved equipment for that. What is important now is not diagnostics, but rather healing itself.' This remark can be interpreted in the same vein as other moves in Nina's general strategy towards biomedical rationale and bureaucratic legitimacy, such as her insistence on the biomedical testing of her patients. Or, it can be seen as the attempt of the charismatic individual to elevate her power over that of inanimate machines: her refusal to waste it on a task that can be addressed by technology.

Be that as it may, her X-ray vision was her password to the semi-medical establishment, and thus to higher reaches of rational-bureaucratic legitimacy. She was accepted on the courses, and, in several months, after getting her certificate as Folk Healer, started work as a resident healer at the centre. She recalls her education fondly, but without much excitement. The trainees listened to lectures on UFOs, on dowsing, and on scientific studies of the 'paranormal'. Nina commented: 'It was fun, but I never related it to myself, to what I had been doing all my life. I do not feel anything paranormal about myself, apart from that time when I acquired distance vision into the life of my lost love.'

About a year later, Nina left the Institute. One reason she gave me was that the general level of the healers practising in the Institute had by then started to deteriorate. 'New people came, and they talked about *szgals* and *porcha*, about some kinship curses that the great grandfather's sins had conferred on the patients, and other such rubbish. Once I heard that a healer in the consulting room next to mine was telling her patient to cure her headache with a hair-curling solution … This was shameful! I could not afford to have my name associated with all these charlatans! After all, I had a medical degree!'

In due time, Nina started her own practice, first with the patients she had come by in the Institute, then expanding it to build the Nina-S centre, her life project and her pride. In spite of all the hardships connected with running a business, this was the way of life she liked most. 'I have always been a leader', she would often say. A strong woman, she managed to build a life for herself in the Russian capital. She was now remarried, and her third husband, the handsome and brawny Valerii, many years her junior, visibly adored her, even as he was afraid to make her angry: she was obviously loved and feared, as the proper Russian empress should be, also by her male favourites.

The time of my fieldwork was a hard one for the clinic and for Nina, but she was never despondent or depressed, and she never entertained so much as a hint of the whinging or 'lamentation and supplication' discourse that, one must admit (*pace* Ries 1997), is not uncommon amongst some in post-Communist Russia. Nor did I ever detect a trace of humility or acceptance of the injustices of fate, as endorsed by the Church and sometimes adopted by religious people. Nina, the charismatic person, obviously rejected the Russian Orthodox virtue of humility in favour of the much castigated vice of pride. Nor did she care about what the Church had to say about her

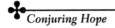

gift and occupation; unlike the majority of people in today's Russia, especially women, she did not acquire any kind of religiosity. If Katerina's self-image was that of a deeply religious person, even though her religiosity was phrased in her own, and not in the Church's terms, Nina presented herself as a pointedly secular person. It was as if she denied the intervention of divine power in her worldly struggles and successes: she had done it all on her own, and she was proud of it.

The only concession she made to mystical higher forces, a notion that she never discussed or defined, the only loophole she left for divine involvement in her activities, was through her hands. As I described above, her hands did their job indexically, through a pantomime of physical corrections to disturbed body tissues. But in her discourse she constructed her hands as 'icons of power', by somehow disengaging them from her self, and endowing them with an agency of their own. She cast her hands as the icons of divine power, while designing her own gestalt in terms of secular power, the power of bureaucratic and rational institutions as well as the strength of character, personality, discipline and will. By doing so, she constructed the secular legitimacy she sought, while retaining the charisma emanating from the same source as other healers lay claim to; the only type of charisma that leads to genuine healing. She never gave it a name, while some called it God, and others were content with labelling it 'the Unknown'.

The Heir of Rasputin

As we have seen, the Nina-S centre was indeed a family enterprise, where family was defined symbolically, broader than in purely kinship terms. It was organised according to one of the paradigmatic models of the Russian family, matriarchally: centred around the figure of a strong and benevolent Little Mother (*Matushka*) Empress, nurturing and hot-tempered, considerate and self-willed. The power of the Empress is so self-evident that it does not need any articulated divine legitimation and can be spelled out in secular terms. However, this model of the matriarchal, extended family leaves room for a male figure, the Empress's favourite, *l'enfant terrible* who dares to break the rules set by the Mother for others, and who is safe from her anger, one that would have rained down on any other of the court vassals for smaller misdemeanours. He is tolerated by virtue of his own personal charisma, which enables him to perform feats of prowess in various domains and thus makes him indispensable. This is a cultural design of charismatic power recognisable, for example, in the historical figure of Potemkin, one of the favourites of Catherine the Great, as well as in that of Rasputin, the healer-monk who cast his spell over the last Empress of Russia, Alexandra, and pushed the Tsar's family towards its violent demise.

At the time of my fieldwork, Georgii was undeniably the main attraction of the Nina-S centre. When the rest of the business was at a low ebb, there were always long lines of patients waiting to be treated by Georgii. This caused Nina some upset, challenging as it did the role of the focal point of the establishment that she reserved for herself. This also made her cherish him, because the Centre was running almost exclusively on the money he earned. Nina and Georgii were old friends; they had met in the Galperin Institute, where Georgii had also obtained his first official 'Folk Healer' certificate.

When I first started my fieldwork at the centre, and still had the status of a guest, Nina used to talk about Georgii exclusively in tones of praise and exultation. According to her, he had a heart of gold; in addition, she called him 'a healer by God's grace', 'really gifted' and 'genuinely powerful'. It seemed that she granted Georgii the same role as she reserved for her own hands: whilst she presented herself as a totally 'normal', 'ordinary' woman, denying everything 'paranormal' or 'other-worldly' in her own endowments and thus ascribing her successes to her own agency, Nina readily accepted Georgii's healing power as emanating from some higher source. Like Nina, but unlike Katerina, Georgii himself in conversation with me never clearly articulated this divine connection. His construction of charisma was through reference to mainly secular, if imaginary and intangible, centres of symbolic power. But whatever his attractiveness derived from, the attraction itself was undeniable and irresistible.

Georgii was a man in his mid-thirties, although he claimed to have turned fifty. This adding of years, instead of the usual strategy of subtracting them, was somewhat idiosyncratic: in Russia as in the West, youth is equated with vitality and potency, and women (though usually not men) spare no efforts to look younger (recall Katerina, whose unimaginably young looks served as evidence of her charismatic power). Men in Russia, especially men of the older generations, usually shun attempts to look younger and more handsome by means of cosmetics; but men, as women, certainly bemoan the passing of the years and the irrevocable loss of youth.

I am not quite sure why Georgii added years to his actual age; perhaps it was in order to indexically aggrandise his own knowledge, wisdom and authority, which in the Russian spiritual tradition is still associated with advanced age, as, for example, is illustrated by the Russian Orthodox tradition of *startsy*.[1] Or, possibly, he wanted to be seen as older in order to accommodate some of the episodes of his personal mythology.

Georgii was of medium height and thick-set, with shoulder-long hair swept back from his balding forehead, a beard that fell onto his wide chest, and a big belly. His face was exceptionally handsome in an icon-like way, with clear and regular features and a grave and piercing gaze. This stern appearance presented a striking contrast to the sudden glances of tenderness and compassion with which he enveloped a patient while listening to his or her story, and also with tender hugs and kisses that he generously bestowed on the female staff of the clinic, which extended to visiting friends as well as to the fieldworking anthropologist. Georgii's 'ecclesiastical' features were lavishly framed in the highest-quality garments of the latest Western fashion, flannel, leather, suede and blue denim in exquisite combinations, which betrayed his sound financial position and keen interest in the world of fashion. A big crucifix on his chest and several massive rings with crosses on his fingers, set with rubies and turquoise in heavy gold settings, completed the picture.

Georgii had the reputation of being a very strong healer. Among his specialties were child cerebral palsy, hormonal growth-deficiency in children, diseases of bones and spine such as osteochandrosis and scoleosis, and also systemic autoimmune diseases. His patients, like those of most healers, were those whom conventional biomedicine had given up. Two patients were always lying on the couches in Georgii's parlour, glass pyramids above their heads, 'for focusing the cosmic energy on their second chakras', as he explained to me. On the walls of the room, acupuncture charts hang next to Russian Orthodox icons, candles and icon-lamps. A stereo tape-recorder played New Age music during the treatment.

Georgii was a trained masseur and taught massage and bone-setting in a nursing school. He had also mastered acupuncture and zone therapy (acupressure), and he prescribed herb mixtures to his patients, claiming to have gathered these himself wandering during summers in the mountains of the Altai, the Urals and Tibet. Most insistently, however, he urged his patients, as part of the treatment, to buy herbal/vitamin/mineral medications produced by the American company called New Ways, an enterprise working in Moscow through pyramidal distribution. Georgii himself was one of the firm's Moscow distributors. Selling these products needed a lot of persuasion, because a bottle of New Ways vitamins cost three times an average monthly salary, and as much as the whole cycle of fifteen treatments by Nina or Georgii himself.

Georgii's séances might include massage and chiropractic treatment for bone and spine diseases; though Georgii no longer did this himself, for there were two other masseurs at the centre. His séances might include acupuncture and acupressure for inflammatory diseases like arthritis or cirrhosis of the liver, but this was all optional. The essence of his treatment, and the only element when he worked with children with cerebral palsy or with systemic diseases like lupus, was the already familiar 'bio-energy treatment'. Unlike all the other healers I ever observed, who usually worked with their hands from a quarter to half an hour, with Georgii this treatment proper took about three minutes. The patient lay on the couch, under the glass pyramid, and Georgii would move his right hand over the ailing parts of the body, or all over the body. These were surgically precise, confident, aesthetically accomplished gestures, but quick as the flutter of a butterfly's wing. As with Nina, they were mimetic movements that iconically represented the operations he performed virtually, in order to smooth out tissues, draw out pus or excise foreign intrusions such as cysts. This performance of healing was a spectacle of some three minutes, that enabled one clearly to see the operation done, with the concrete sequence of healing procedures perfectly embodied in the act.

The strange thing, however, was that the observing anthropologist was the only, and very rare, spectator, because the patient always lay with her eyes closed. Other possible spectators might be a child's mother or a patient's next of kin, but this was far from always the case. The pantomime theatre of Georgii (and other healers like him) is not meant for spectators, being in many cases a one-man theatre. After this quick performance Georgii lit a candle on the wall in front of one of the icons (the icon-lamp, *lampada*, was always burning, as is the tradition in Russian Orthodox households), put on New Age music, and left: to attend to another patient, to answer the telephone, to chat with the staff who solved crosswords in the waiting room, or to disappear with one of his many young female admirers who were often in attendance waiting for this moment.

When I asked Georgii why his treatment took such a short time, he explained somewhat vaguely that with his fast movements he set into operation a curing programme within the bio-energy-information field of the patient. He also told me that while he was chatting with me or doing something else, part of his mind was with the patient, incessantly continuing the healing work. He also said that he actually knew exactly what the patient was doing there lying on the couch, what she was feeling, if the pain was stronger or weaker, if she stirred, scratched herself, or coughed. Nor did he even need to look at his watch in order to know it was time to release the patient.

I was first introduced to Georgii as a Swedish researcher writing a book on healers. He was polite in a dry and austere way, displaying an attitude of authority and distance coupled with a focused gaze and undivided attention that gave you the impression that he looked right through you and knew the secrets of your body and soul. This was Georgii's mode of behaviour with strangers, with actual and potential patients. It soon gave way to a more casual and cuddly stance that he maintained with more stable connections, friends and acquaintances, as well as with the staff of the centre: warm and broad-armed embraces and tender kisses on lips and cheeks that stopped just short of being too long to be purely friendly.

At our first conversation, when he heard that I was from Sweden, he said: 'Actually, I have Swedish roots. My mother comes from a very rich Swedish family. She died when she gave birth to me, and my father was arrested by the KGB a week before I was born. I don't remember my mother, but I have her photograph, with a note: "To my little sunshine, my beloved son". Later in life, I found my mother's relatives in Sweden, and I even went to Stockholm to meet them. But they were not nice to me: perhaps they thought that I would claim my share of the family fortune. I decided never to see them again; so, I won't go to Sweden any more.'

Later he told me that he had three academic degrees, and that he used to be fluent in four foreign languages. But he decided to take a break in his academic career and enrolled in an elite paratrooper regiment. He was sent to Vietnam, became shell-shocked there, and lost his foreign languages. One consequence of the shell-shock was that he lost the ability to learn languages at all. 'My first teacher was Baturin, a famous Russian healer then living in Tashkent, the founder of a chiropractics and osteopathy school [and a promoter of Tibetan medicine]. I got interested in massage and bone-setting when I went through his treatment myself, convalescing after the shell-shock. When I watched how the masseur worked, I realised this was what I wanted to do. I went to Baturin and asked him to accept me as his student. He looked at me and said: "You don't need to be my student, you are already better at this than myself. You are a born healer." Still, I was his apprentice for a number of years.'

'But my first real teacher was a Tibetan monk. I met him in Tashkent: I was walking in an empty street in the old city, at dusk. I saw this man in his bright orange robe passing by. And then a group of young thugs appeared from behind a wall and surrounded him, asking for money. I rushed up and, to protect him, started to fight with them, but he silently gestured to me to stop. He made an almost imperceptible movement with his hand, and three of them were down on the ground, writhing with pain. The other two ran away. "Follow me", he said to me in pure Russian (as it turned out later, he was from Buryatiya), "I see that you have a gift. Nobody can teach you the art of healing, but stay with me if you wish, and I shall pass my knowledge on to you". I spent three years in Tibet with him, learning bone-setting and herbal remedies. He taught me to touch patients, listen, and ask questions, and be more precise in my diagnosing. But nobody can teach you to heal. You are born with the gift, but it comes forth gradually. I stayed with him for three years, and then he said: "Now you are ready to leave: you know all I know." Then I studied with sorcerers in Iran and with shamans in Siberia. It was the same story with them: they always decided when my apprenticeship with them was done and I was ready to go.'

'My next personal teacher after my Tibetan guru was an old wise woman [*babka* or *babushka*] from Briansk [a forest area in middle Russia]. Baba Nastia lived in a tiny hut deep in the forest with her sister who helped her with herbs and with the household chores.

Patients came to her themselves, she was known far and wide. When I first went to see her, she was very stern with me. I had to sweep her yard and scour her pots for six months, and only watched from a distance how she treated her patients. Once her dog hurt its paw, and baba Nastia saw me heal it. Then she told me: "Come in now. I shall show you how to heal." I stayed with her for about a year. She taught me a lot about bone-setting and herbs. Many diseases can be healed by bone-setting to begin with. Everything starts from the spine. And in the end she also told me: "You are ready to go and work on your own. I have taught you all I know."'

Once I remarked on his crucifix, and he told me that he also was a priest, ordained by a Greek Orthodox bishop somewhere in a remote monastery in Greece. 'He gave me the crucifix as a sign that I was ordained', he said.

A Russian colleague-ethnologist had worked with both Nina and Georgii before, and both of them have long since been among her favourite informants and study objects. They agreed to cooperate in the laboratory, when their abilities were being tested with technical equipment. They also told their stories on her tape recorder, and gave her healing if the need arose. My colleague thought it would be interesting to compare notes about the various parts of Georgii's fantastic biography. She told me with a laugh that the 'Swedish part' came up especially in my honour, whereas the rest of it she had already heard before. On another occasion, she tried to interview him for an article she was working on, and she started to probe him on the specifics of the Siberian shamans that he claimed had been amongst his teachers. At that point he became reticent and even a bit upset and said that this information was secret, and that he should probably reconsider the generosity with which he always allowed people to interview him. In a word, and not surprisingly, when he sensed incredulity and ridicule, he closed up.

At some point in my interaction with Georgii, Nina, informed by her spies, told me with a smile: 'Do I surmise correctly that you have been treated to the adventures of our Professor? He has a heart of gold and magical hands, but you should take his stories with a grain of salt. This one about the Vietnam war – it could never be true, he is just thirty-six years old! He had a bad childhood, poor guy! He never had a proper family: his father had abandoned his mother before he was born, she was a drunkard and burned their house down when he was a child. He grew up in an orphanage. His training with the Gurus, that's all rubbish! He was actually educated as a masseur, in a nursing school, apart from the Galperin Institute, and that's all the degrees he has. Massage is what he teaches in a nursing school now. It's funny when he introduces himself to people as Professor! He has this tremendous need for self-aggrandizement. I'm not at all like this myself … I am a simple woman and I am not ashamed of it!'

Later I was invited to a show in the nursing school where Georgii was employed as a teacher. I never found out whether he taught massage, as Nina claimed, or general anatomy and pharmaceutical science, as was his version. What was clear, however, was that Georgii enjoyed enormous popularity among the almost all-female population of the nursing school. Not only did he teach there; he also led a drama group and was a stage director of amateur theatre shows that the school put on annually, as part of a contest to determine the 'Nurse with the Golden Hands'. He also composed songs, both lyrics and music, and performed them on stage, in a deep baritone voice, and with brilliant artistry: he could as well have been an opera singer or a Russian Orthodox priest, another vocation that needs good singing skills. His success in the show was overwhelming: the audience burst into tempestuous applause, screamed 'More, more!', as if he were a rock star. The man's charisma was strong enough to gather crowds of followers; he told me, however, that healing was the only thing he really loved – singing was second best, and he would have never traded one for the other. 'It is my gift, my mission,' he told me, 'This is what God wants me to do, and I shall do it, even if I don't get any money for it.'

After the show a small celebration ensued at the premises of the Centre. Several girls joined us; I had seen them before, sitting discreetly in the waiting room. Nina treated them with her usual benevolence, but to me she characterised them snidely as 'our Professor's ladies-in-waiting'. The composition of the group changed over the years, but the phenomenon remained, she said: they were like a cloud of small stick-fish around a big shark. They came from his students, his former patients, and the members of his drama groups. They sat for hours, waiting for Georgii to come out of his consulting room, to catch a glimpse of him, maybe to talk to him; sometimes he disappeared with some of them out of sight for half an hour, or they would follow him home. Otherwise, the girls chatted with the staff, discussing fashions and recipes, or doing crosswords; it was as if they were tacitly considered part of the extended family of the Nina-S. Some disappeared, but they would be replaced with new ones. During a later visit Nina caustically informed me that Georgii had landed a really rich one. She gave him a mobile phone as a present, real kudos in Moscow at those times (though not in 2003 as I write). The staff was thus deprived of the pleasure of eavesdropping on Georgii's private conversations, which they otherwise enjoyed immensely, exchanging meaningful glances and giggling to themselves.

Only once did I manage to have Georgii all to myself (not counting semi-formal interviews in the presence of my ethnologist-friend, and hasty exchanges in between his treatments): I invited him for dinner, and he gladly accepted. Our private conversation acquired an unexpected, although familiar tone, in the well-known genre of lamentation (Ries 1997) (otherwise absent in the centre). The charismatic Rasputin figure suddenly turned into a miserable little boy, in need of comfort and consolation. He told me about the difficulties of working in the centre, about the lack of respect he was experiencing from Nina and the staff, about the need to pay for the apartment he had bought on borrowed money and about his lack of money, since only half of what he earned was going to his own pocket. He told me about his failed family life: his wife, a stage actress, had left him and taken away their son, whom Georgii adored and always talked proudly about as a little boy with fabulous healing (and other) abilities. Georgii missed his son enormously, he confessed; but he did not miss his wife, because he did not love her; in fact, it was his previous wife who was the love of his life, but she died in a car crash when she was three months pregnant. This episode of Georgii's biography was also new for those who had known him longer than I; invented or not, it was obviously narrated in order to reinforce the air of tragedy and suffering. It was merely one element of the 'Tragic Hero' persona, a key that certainly had the capacity to open up (some) Russian selves; to unlock some, especially female, hearts.

We can see, then, that both Nina and Georgii construct themselves, albeit perhaps unconsciously, as icons of power in different, though comparable ways. In their narratives and styles of behaviour, they employ various legitimation strategies, discernible in the way other Russian healers and magi present themselves. There are references to the 'symbolic centres of power and vitality' valued by society at large. There are also more subtle and more general paradigmatic cultural designs, that appeal, not to the cognitive and symbolic, but to the aesthetic and emotional sensibilities of their fellow citizens. Nina's image is that of a Matriarch, a strong woman recognisable from other practitioners of the craft. She is both the Lover and the Mother, both a sensual and attractive woman and a keen politician and strategist, a warrior where it takes a fight, an attentive and nourishing consoler when those weaker come to her for help. In her discourse, the divine as the source of her charisma is underarticulated. It is partly transferred from Heaven to Society, but ultimately to her own self, and even more specifically, to a certain part of her body, namely, her hands.

Georgii, a healer-lover-monk, opens hearts as a figure with spiritual endowments, as well as a man with secular talents that are invested with high social acclaim (such as his stage directing and singing talents). His attraction is augmented by the appeal to people's (especially women's) predilection for empathy and compassion for the kind but ill-understood, the deserving but unhappy: he is both the saviour and the one to be salvaged. At the same time, Georgii is consistent in maintaining that the source of his charisma is not of this world: a gift that cannot be taught, that can only be received through divine grace.

Nina forges legitimacy by reference to an authoritative system: that of biomedical knowledge. Although she is proud of her village roots, the Russian tradition as the source of legitimacy is in her discourse clearly understated. Still, the area of her reference is distinctly local: the world beyond Russia does not even appear in her stories. Georgii, on the contrary, creates his image as a man of knowledge by referring to a version of the global world that is partly culturally shared, and partly individually created. His version of the globe brings to mind the map that, as Boym wrote, was familiar to those living in Russia in Stalin's times: 'the multinational Soviet Union with Moscow as its geographical centre and the centre of ideological gravity' (1994: 114). The USSR, one-fifth of the land-mass of the globe, was a metonym for the entire world, just as Russia was a metonym for the Soviet Union, despite the rhetoric of the multinational state in use at those times. Somewhere on the other side of the world there was the USA – an evil counterbalance to the good that Russia represented. Clearly, the USA is also a source of fascination for Georgii, as it is for many of his compatriots, as his paratrooper story and his purported involvement in Vietnam indicate. Yet for him the USA is also a place of loss, since he loses his four foreign languages because of the Vietnam war, and thus severs his symbolic connection with the North American and European world. The route from Russia out into the Western world is thus closed to Georgii; all his other global pathways are from the outside and in. His present involvement with America, his connection with the natural medicine company 'New Ways', is a purely pragmatic undertaking, not a source of learning, not an input into his knowledge and healing art, but a materialistic supplement to his healing, since it represents, also pragmatically, a source of monetary income.

Affiliation with the Church is another legitimating strategy that Georgii uses in his mythopoesis (while Nina never so much as mentions the Church). As transpires from the advertisements mentioned in Chapter 1, this is a strategy he shares with many other healers. But his Orthodoxy is not Russian, which, in many people's view, is corrupted, opportunistic, conservative, and connected with the darker political forces of xenophobic nationalism. Instead, Georgii's religiousness comes from Russia's spiritual precursor, Orthodox Greece, from the rural, ascetic, monastic tradition. Real knowledge, the silver dove of wisdom, comes from the pure springs of the East – a Tibetan Lama (though speaking perfect Russian), Persian wizards, Siberian shamans. This is the legitimacy of non-Western traditions, the attraction of the exotic. Traditional legitimacy is also drawn from the depths of the domestic Russian tradition, embodied in the mythic figure of a little *bábushka* hiding away in a hut in the thick of the Russian woods, bringing to mind the sorceress baba Yaga of Russian folk tales. Georgii's global world consists of realms south-east of the Caucasus, all flowing from the outside and in. These are his sources of wisdom, to be ignited and fertilised by the spark of Russian folk tradition, grounded by Russian roots.

Nina and Georgii were two people who struggled in post-Soviet Moscow to act as icons of power in order to heal others, but also to live their versions of good and worthy lives. Theirs was a battle on unequal conditions: these people had nothing going for them from

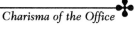

the outsets of their biographies, except for their strange gift, their personal strength that they tried to frame through salient cultural designs, to perpetuate it. Propped up by this scaffolding, they survived day by day, until they perished, crushed by more merciless structures. When I returned to Moscow in 2002, the Nina-S centre was closed. I never found out what happened: Nina's home telephone did not answer; maybe her landlords had done a raid on her (*naekhali*), and she had had to move. Maybe the centre was closed because it had been abandoned by Georgii, who had disappeared to the USA: he was invited to work there and stayed there for a year or two. Later, I heard that Georgii finally did come back: maybe he did not want to stay in the USA, unable to learn the language, whether or not as a consequence of his shell-shock trauma. Thus, America did lure the post-Soviet Rasputin, only to spit him out later. I lost track of both of them; I would like to think that they are well, not just managing, but continuing as persons of charisma, giving away in healing the power that is gratefully received by others.

Concluding digression: iconicity of power in Russia

In this and the previous chapter, I presented three individuals who earn their living through offering healing to others. They can do so because they are recognised by their fellow citizens as charismatic individuals, as people with a special, perhaps divine, gift that is understood to exceed ordinary human sensory abilities, and that can be expressed in the power of their consciousness (or their hands) to transform the ailing matter of others' bodies and environments in favourable directions. By referring to them as 'icons of power', I did not mean to say that they consciously construct themselves as certain cultural archetypes. It is rather that through being the way they are, they partake in 'culturally envisaged sources of fundamental power or vital force' (Geertz 1977), and are seen by some people as 'desirable' (their clients, according to their own confession, 'fall in love' with them, as many female patients of Georgii testify). Being appealing, coming forth as 'desirable', these people are conceived by others as imbued with 'power and vital force', and so they can iconically transfer this power in healing.

In the Introduction I quoted Roy Rappaport (1999) who in his last magisterial work argues that the divine power is always manifested for the faithful through iconic and indexical modes of signification. The question remains, however: how is it possible that these mundane people are so easily recognised as bearers (or icons) of the divine power? How are the minor miracles that their clients perceive them to achieve integrated so easily into the latter's picture of the world?

Probably this becomes understandable if we think of the place that Russian Orthodox icons (*ikony*) occupied in everyday life all through Russian history (and they are strongly coming back again now). Icon-painting has been for centuries the only existing type of painting in Russia, where creativity of painters was at one with their religious ardour. The images on the icons were not *representations* of the Divine, but were considered to be its *presentations*, the essence of the Divine itself, a direct door to Heaven and an incarnate manifestation of Heaven in material form. An icon brought, for the faithful, the Sacred into the midst of the mundane world, thus making the divine essence, pragmatically, part of the mundane. The long tradition of miracle-working icons, which has been revived in present-day Russia, is a manifestation of this domestication of the agency of the divine power. For the faithful, healing was effectuated through direct contact with the source of this power (and, of course, other Christian traditions, too, have miracle-working objects and sites of pilgrimage).

The earthly power of the Soviet era set out to destroy religious institutions, but structured itself as a divine power, offering the grand promise of salvation (impending Communism), and crafting its leaders as divinities on earth. It is not inimical to Russian structures of selfhood to worship earthly powers as if they were divine ones (see Berdyaev 1990). Before the revolution, the tradition of pilgrimage to miracle-working icons, relics of saints and elderly healer-monks (*startsy*) enabled people to partake in the heavenly power manifested iconically. By the same token, in Soviet times, thousands of people from all over the empire stood in line for hours in order to pass by the embalmed body of Lenin, the central icon of the power that structured their lives.

The innumerable images of Lenin flooded the public space: from kindergartens to workplaces, from art galleries and entertainment locales to the places where life-cycle rituals took place, signifying nothing else than the all-pervasiveness, the ubiquity of power. At parades twice a year, smaller, living icons of power stood atop of the mausoleum in Red Square. Faceless and indistinguishable from each other, they represented nothing, but iconically presented power in its superhuman grandeur. In contrast to the healers described above, they were icons of power not because they were appealing and desirable, but because they, in a different way, were connected with the source of the mundane state power. In contrast to healers, their 'significant effect' (the effect of their 'presentation') was not to heal, but to hold people in the grips of power: to remind them of its eternal and naturalised character.

Thus, the signs of power in Russia have always been more presentational than representational. They were more iconic and indexical, working by dint of the knowledge of *how* they signify, than symbolic, based on cognitively achieved consensus of rational interpretation. Therefore, these icons of power could be put to different kinds of pragmatic work: their purport, as Peirce would put it, lay not in their meaning, but in their bearing on the conduct of life.

Note

1. *Startsy* were old wise men, who lived in Russian Orthodox monasteries and were treated as saints while they were still alive. Their saintliness, coupled with the exceptional austerity of their way of life and often with an extreme severity of attitude, was expressed in their wisdom, and, not least, in their power to heal. There are still renowned *startsy* in contemporary Russian Orthodox monasteries, people who stand out as centres of authority and power in their own right, attracting both pilgrims and disciples.

Chapter 6
The Unspeakable Emotions: Spells and Their Use in Working Life

There is a long tradition of studying magical language in anthropology, starting from Malinowski (1922, 1965) and continuing through Lévi-Strauss (1963) and Stanley Tambiah (1968, 1990) to Thomas Csordas (1997a) (to name but a few). There are two main ideas that have transpired in this scholarship that are relevant to my argument below. One is that all rhetoric and ritual language, spells included, is more instrumental than expressive, or, more precisely, that in this kind of language these two aspects are indistinguishable. In the Peircian terms adopted in this book, ritual speech is more pragmatic than descriptive or referential, and, thus, it acts, primarily, iconically and indexically.

The other is the idea that rhetoric speech, including spells, offers ways to manipulate the subjectivity of the speaker (and the audience) and, according to Csordas (ibid.), to create new subjective and intersubjective realities. In this chapter, I shall regard spells of Russian magic as means to 'restructure and integrate the minds and emotions of the actors' (Tambiah 1968: 202), but I shall take a somewhat different tack. I shall consider spells as 'icons of power', that is, entities that are culturally conceived to have some kind of affinity (or, as Peirce puts it, 'community') in structure, quality or appearance with the existing clusters of power. In so doing, I shall take another look at what this power is about, on its grids and ontologies. I shall try to see what the spells of Russian magic can tell us about the subjectivity of those who use them, and about the power structures of the domains in which they are used.

170

The use of words placed together in specially arranged patterns has been an essential element of magical practice in many cultures and in many historical times.[1] Scientifically inclined Russian folklorists note this fact and offer an explanation: when uttered, patterned strings and clusters of words occasion vibrations of air on certain frequencies. These interact with the human brain and body, transforming it and thus achieving their healing or harming effect.[2] Katerina's explanation is of a similar kind: according to her, spells are programmed energy patterns, which, when uttered and accompanied by the requisite ritual actions, change the energy-information structures of the world and alter its physical and situational patterns in desired directions.

Katerina's reasoning in favour of the effectiveness of spells is that they exist because they have been used for centuries; and they have been used because they work – otherwise, why should they exist? This reasoning corresponds to the argument put forward by Malinowski in his studies of Trobriand spells, as well as to that suggested by Lévi-Strauss in 'The Effectiveness of Symbols' (1963): the power of magic is inextricably linked to the warrant of tradition (Malinowski 1922: 400); the force of the spell is derived from the knowledge that the words uttered have roots in history. Katerina's remark also points to the element of 'belief' that underlies the efficacy of magic tools: like all magic and other metaphysical healing, they work because they are expected to work. This is a well-known line of argument deployed in the anthropology of healing ever since Malinowski and Lévi-Strauss, and summarised in the 'intellectualist' approach outlined by Skorupski (1976). The patient feels differently because she is made to think differently, and this change of thinking is predicated on the force of faith; healing works because such acts have worked before and because they are expected to work. This 'placebo effect theory', however, calls for further exploration of the specific logic of its efficacy.

When uttered, spells are understood to act as 'icons of power' – to change reality, to alter the situation, be it ailments of body or the unsatisfactory situational configurations in interpersonal relations, business, trade and working life. Dynamics of signification of these various semiotic 'bullets' or 'missiles'[3] – or 'magic darts', as known from classical shamanism – must be homologous to that of larger patterns of power dynamics. In the previous chapters, I have considered a number of such units of potency: specific notions, as in terms of affliction, gestural performance, as in the pantomime of healing, and simple rituals such as reading away with prayers or rolling off with eggs. Furthermore, as I have tried to show, the figures of power, magi themselves, can as well be seen as icons of power.

Bourdieu's maxim states that the logic of practice is not that of a logician. As Sartre (1976) argues in his 'Phenomenology of Emotions', the logic of emotions is not that of a logician either. Instead, the existential attitude of the impassioned self to the object of passion (and to the surrounding world) strongly resembles the ways of handling the world that are known as magical. Spells are passions condensed; emotions cast into proper poetic form that the culture provided through generations, out of the blood, sweat and tears of ancestors who struggled with the same predicaments, who were plagued by the same passions[4]. People use these verbal missiles, the containers of meaning, because what these poetic pieces say conveys 'the grammar of affects' – the deep phenomenological patterns of their states of 'body, soul and spirit' – better than other, freely chosen words.

Setting aside questions of vibrations and structures of the 'thin planes' (*tonkie plany*, or energo-information fields), one thing is indisputable: people use spells because they resonate with their immediate experiences and agendas, and because they package and congeal their own affects and intentionalities in evocative and poetically expressive ways. Spells are jewels of social poetics, which both endow human passions with a form perfected over centuries, and legitimate these passions by stating that they are integral to core cultural patterns of sociality, inasmuch as they have survived political transformations, technological innovations and social turmoil. Ontologies of power, the relational dynamics between the agents, are always in motion, shifting, uncertain, and difficult to grasp; but they are still patterned in certain ways, guiding and limiting people's imagination of the possible and the desirable. Spells work indexically as icons of power because the relational dynamics they convey are homologous with those that pertain to the situations in which they are used. Therefore, the texts of spells must betray the deep underlying dynamics of power and sociality that are discursively underdeveloped, but that are at the core of attitudes and values that steer everyday life, and mould and modify the imported and newly generated institutions into practices that are people's own: both recognisable and culturally distinctive.

In Russian magical practice, there are spells to deal with all of life's conceivable misfortunes. There are spells for failures in love as well as in other close bonds of sociality. These are bonds that are supposed to be bearing for the individual, but that in reality turn out to undermine or destroy her existence, such as those with the mother-in-law and other kin. There are spells to sever the bonds that are conceived as life-sustaining but turn out to be destructive, such as the spell to force the husband to let his wife go and to grant her a divorce. There are spells to cure various diseases and disturbances of health, like arthritis, kidney stones, mental disorders and epilepsy. A large corpus of spells deals with sexual and reproductive problems. Spells against impotence and sterility (and rituals connected with them) are a category on their own; there are spells pertaining to pregnancy, children's health and other aspects of child-rearing (more on spells in Russian magic is found in Ryan 1999).

Another special category of spells is used in working life: in small- and medium-size businesses, in business transactions such as buying and selling, and at workplaces in salaried jobs. As Katerina sees it, all sorts of business are ultimately about interpersonal relations, and business transactions are hugely impacted by the human 'intensities' of these relational dynamics. This, according to her, is especially true for small and medium business (less so for the big ones, although they operate according to similar laws), and it is this chemistry of intersubjectivity that the spells are designed to alter. There are spells for dealing with business partners, competitors, potential and real enemies, with those who 'make raids on you' (*naezzhat'*), trying to deprive you of live-sustaining energy in the forms of money and working space. There are spells against those who try to 'throw' you on money, and against those who extort money from you, putting you 'on the counter' when the days of your life start ticking away. There are spells used in dealings with superiors and other co-workers, whose antipathy can cost you your livelihood, in the absence of any legal mechanisms to secure your job. If the spells are congealed passions, they can be semiotically considered as Representamina to the emotions that they bespeak and that they try to manipulate. Therefore, the texts of these spells can tell us much about the nature of these emotions.

The spells are composed in the archaic language[5] of the disadvantaged and the disempowered of previous centuries: merchants who sold their goods from stalls in markets in villages or small towns; peasants in serfdom, hired farm hands, menial workers of the early era of urbanisation and industrialisation. The archaicity and the low-class provenance of the language of spells account for much of their expressive power. Without embarrassment, they mix the appeals to God, God's Mother, Christ, and the Archangels, with sexual and scatological obscenities; and the language of prayer with that of secular supplication and mundane curse. The words are antiquated, known only from bygone folklore. The archaicity of the language, the use of colloquial and even foul words next to those from devout or pious discourse, mark the poetics of spells, and account for their expressive effectiveness. Some of this is lost in translation; what is conveyed in the texts below are the bare bones of the meaning of the spells. But, after all, apart from their poetic and entertaining value it is the structure of meaning of the spells that makes for their efficacy.

Spells are but one of the elements of magical treatment, in no way indispensable, and used only by certain types of magi with certain types of clients. The archaic and rural provenance of spells must logically limit their use to those clients who can take seriously the expressive arsenal of village folk culture. It would be difficult for me to imagine a representative of urban technical intelligentsia, with no roots in the village, reciting Russian magic spells other than jestingly. But then, again, it all depends on the degree of the severity of the predicament: who knows what a person would resort to being stripped of any other hope? In the cases below, the users of spells are young, educated urbanites in the middle of their upward mobility course. I imagine they, and others, were embarrassed to be uttering spells, even silently, and took great care to make their use of spells strictly private. This is perhaps the reason why one of them, Dmitrii, was in denial regarding the impact of spells in one particular instance of his business activities. This is also why I never discussed the use of spells with the users themselves – this was one of the subjects on which most of them invariably turned reticent. What did they feel when they murmured to themselves these burning, charged words? I shall never know. The subjectivity of the users can be surmised only from the poetry of the spells themselves. However, in order to convey the context in which spells are used, below are two cases from Katerina's practice where spells played a prominent role. Both these cases were narrated to me by Katerina herself. The protagonist of the first of them, Anna, had disappeared from the circle of Katerina's clients; the second, Dmitrii, was still a regular client and had great respect for Katerina, but he would never discuss his treatment with me, much less admit that any spells were used.

Anna, in her late twenties, was pretty and attractive. In Katerina's words, she made one think of rising dough about to spill out of its container: her full and round forms seemed a little bit too big for the size of the clothes she wore. But Anna was not concerned with weight-watching; on the contrary, she was proud of her voluptuous shape and aware of her good looks. She was also clever. She had graduated from a prestigious medical college with high grades, and she found herself a good job as a therapist in a private medical clinic. This was a clinic for people with money, and Anna's salary, some 700 dollars, was about twice the average family income, which was quite respectable for a young, recently graduated doctor. Anna had a sharp tongue, and she never hesitated to snap at those who were cutting up rough, and to talk back, no matter what the status of the interlocutor was. She was a proud woman with a temper, and she was not going to allow anyone to step on her tail, as the Russian saying goes; this, of course, often got her in trouble. She came to Katerina with a common problem: she could not get herself a life partner. Men were attracted to her sexually, and many had already passed through her life, but none of them stayed; either they left themselves, repelled by her independent and catty disposition, or she discarded them, because she found that they were 'parasites' with nothing to give.

Katerina's diagnosis was 'a karmic problem'. This, in her terminology, means a fundamental flaw in a person's character that makes her time and again make the wrong decisions of the same kind. The consequences of such decisions are invariably detrimental to the person, and their gravity increases with every successive round; but, as if wired by a program, this kind of person makes the same mistakes and puts herself in the same situations. In Katerina's definition, the karmic problem is the root of 'karmic knots': situations caused and conditioned by the person's karmic problems, which corner her into taking radical decisions. When faced with a karmic knot, the person should first realise what the wrong patterns are, and then start to behave differently, change her own rutted behaviour patterns and thus the responses of the environment.

Anna's karmic problem was that she made too high demands on life and had unrealistically high expectations. This is often the essence of Katerina's message to women who come to her complaining that they can not find their 'Prince'. As she said to me, 'They want someone who is young and handsome, who earns good money and will take care of them materially, and who is sensitive and emotionally in tune with their souls' needs ... and who is great in bed, and at the same time faithful only to them ... But those things are mutually exclusive!'

Katerina started séances with Anna, monitoring her behaviour throughout in concrete situations, with potential suitors and admirers and with other people she encountered in life. Among other things, Katerina tried to convince Anna to curb her sharp tongue and to stop telling people exactly what she thought of their physical and mental flaws. This was especially counter-productive with Anna's boss in the clinic, a woman somewhat older than Anna, but also in her best years, 'good-looking but dried-up, like a herring', as Anna characterised her, and, also according to Anna's information, totally alone in life. According to Anna, her female boss detested her success with men, the success that she herself lacked. According to Katerina, the boss disliked Anna's way of cheekily answering back, especially when she was quite rightly reproached, as, for example, for her bad habit of always coming to work late. 'Yes, she [Anna] had this total lack of reliability (*neobiazatel'nost'*),' commented Katerina, 'She would also come late to our séances, forty minutes late, and she was not even embarrassed about it – another manifestation of her karmic problem.'

Anna was troubled by her relations with her boss. Bosses, everywhere, have many ways of making life miserable for their subordinates. In Russia, now as before, bosses are often sole rulers with unlimited authority. Should Anna's boss decide so, Anna would be fired there and then, without either any discussion or payment. To be fired was a nightmare for Anna, not only because this was a dream job for her, but also because she badly needed money to pay for the care of her bedridden mother paralysed after a stroke. Katerina considered that the problem with the boss was partly due to Anna's karmic problem, that is, her bad attitude and her sharp tongue. This was treated 'energy-wise', through Katerina's séances. It was also monitored through their conversations, which took place daily by telephone, where Anna briefed Katerina on what had happened during the day on the battlefield that Anna's workplace had became, to receive concrete advice as to how to do better. Additionally, the 'karmic problem' was treated with a variety of spells, applied according to the 'schema' that Katerina had devised.

These spells were read over water by Katerina herself, and Anna was instructed to wash her face and hands with this water at certain times of the day, early in the morning and once more before going to work. She was also advised to take the water to her clinic and furtively, in the bathroom, wash her face with it, saying the spell to herself. Another spell was given to Anna to read over water, to bring this water to her office and to leave it hidden under her desk. All these measures started to bear fruit; the boss seemed to be kinder to Anna, and, at a party after a little alcohol she even drew Anna aside and tried to talk to her 'as a human being': 'well, you understand that you really can't behave this way ... I have nothing against you personally, but ...' Both Anna and Katerina thought things were going right, when the crisis came.

Anna called Katerina in tears, to tell her that she had been fired. It happened one Tuesday morning when she came to work forty minutes late, as sometimes happened. Her boss was the first person she ran into in the corridor of the clinic, and, when confronted, Anna answered in all honesty that she had overslept: she just had not heard her alarm clock ring. The boss grew furious and said that Anna was fired, as of the coming Monday. Katerina told Anna to keep her cool, saying that there were still several days to Monday, during which time much can happen. That was time to move in the heavy artillery, as Katerina put it to me. She gave Anna a special prayer, *molitva zaderzhaniia*. *Zaderzhat'* is to detain, to keep waiting, or to keep someone engaged in a conversation or some other activities, thus preventing one from doing something else. *Zaderzhat'* also means to halt the march of the troops, the approach or the attack of the enemy in the field. In today's magical world of Russia, this prayer is used as a last resort, to stop the inevitable approach of something threatening, some superior brute force rolling over you and about to crush you mercilessly. It is used, among other things, against *'naezdy'* (a new Russian slang word explained above).

Katerina told me that the prayer of *zaderzhanie* is considered to be an extremely strong prayer, to be used in situations where all other means have been exhausted, and only very few old prayer books contain it. To use it, devout Orthodox Christians have to ask for special permission from their priest or spiritual father. It appeals for the help of selected Russian saints, Archangels and Our Lady, and invokes martyrs and spiritual heroes whose inevitable demise was diverted through the intervention of higher forces. Katerina instructed Anna to read this prayer once a day, first thing in the morning, while she herself worked on the situation 'energy-wise', through her own channels, as she put it. During the four days that were left for Anna at her job, the boss never got to write the official firing order. On Monday it turned out that the boss herself was fired, replaced by a male colleague from the same clinic who was Anna's friend and patron, and who had helped her to find this job in the first place. With this man as her boss, Anna's job was secured beyond any doubt. She never thanked Katerina for that, however. 'As all of them, she took it for granted', Katerina remarked.

Instead, in a couple of weeks, Anna called Katerina, complaining of another crisis, this time of a personal nature. The man with whom she thought she was developing a real relationship, the man who had rented an apartment for them to live together in, with whom she was planning to move in with, suddenly told her that he did not want her anymore. Katerina tried to find out what had caused it, what events had preceded this breakdown. Anna was adamant that it had all come out of the blue, that absolutely nothing had happened between them. ('You understand, of course, that this is impossible, that such things do not happen all by themselves. People lie so much …', Katerina commented.) 'If you don't want to tell me the truth, there is not much I can do about it', said Katerina to Anna. That was the end of their contact; Anna never turned to Katerina again. 'She never paid me the hundred dollars she owed me for the last séances', was Katerina's impassioned summary of the story.

Dmitrii's father was a minister during Soviet times, so Dmitrii grew up as a member of the gilded youth, not needing to worry about anything. He did not receive any college education, and during Soviet years and well into perestroika he earned his living as a professional card-player. At some point he decided that this occupation was taking too heavy a toll on his nerves, and quit. He started to build houses, and had made a tidy sum on the deal. He had inherited good contacts from his father, some of whom had been nomenklatura before and had since become New Russians. He used this social capital to buy a big apartment in an elite gated community outside Moscow, and to become a chief engineer, responsible for the utility maintenance in the area. Through this activity he multiplied his fortune, and he developed sufficient contacts to receive orders to build houses for New Russians (see Humphrey 2002b, Chapter 9), the famous villas outside Moscow that look so strange, but that sell so well when they do sell.

At the time he came to Katerina, Dmitrii was in his mid-forties, a good-looking man with money and charm, but with his health totally ruined. He suffered from phobias, fears of closed spaces and crowded streets, he was frightened to fly, and he had difficulties sleeping. He was plagued by aches all over his body, and obtained diagnoses from various doctors in expensive private clinics. The last of them was necrosis of the kidney, and the doctors told him that he would die in two years' time. He himself also felt that his days were numbered, and he was suffocated by the fear of death. He had visited a number of magi and healers in Moscow, but he did not feel they had helped. His business went well, he was making money, but he was constantly consumed with pain and fear. This was when he met Katerina.

Katerina saw that Dmitrii had a rare gift that she called 'the realisation channel'. This meant that he implemented whatever plans and visions he had in life; he was also a strong-willed person, capable of shaping his 'lived-in space' (*zhiznennoie prostranstvo*) according to his designs. Katerina also diagnosed a very heavy *porcha* on Dmitrii. She traced this *porcha* to the times when he worked as the chief engineer of the utility service in the elite gated community outside Moscow. She suggested that he had made some less than honest transactions that brought him big money but that had angered certain individuals. She saw that some people worked on him magically, to do him in. He readily admitted that this was exactly the case. Katerina told him that his *porcha* was so grave and worked on him so strongly because his own sensitivity was so high, and he was in touch with 'the thin plane'. In other words, Dmitrii had some extrasensory or magical abilities himself, but he had never worked to develop them, and never engaged in any spiritual activities. He admitted that this was true: when he was growing up, his environment was far from spiritual, and when he matured and discovered that 'these things' indeed attracted him, he had no time for them, since he was busy making money. Katerina also saw some ruined love, a rejected woman who had worked magically to hurt Dmitrii, but this he definitively denied: he was not interested in women, he was quite content with his wife, who was small, thin, and very quiet. Katerina asked if there was any problem with the wife. Dmitrii did not see any problem, and if there was, he was always able to solve it himself. His wife used to drink heavily and to get into trouble, and so Dmitrii had to take her away from her work. Now she was staying home, saying nothing, doing nothing, just smoking silently. But she did not demand anything from her husband, and she did not make scenes, so he thought their life worked quite well.

Dmitrii was one of the most convincing successes in Katerina's practice. His phobias went away after a month of her séances, he stopped taking medication, he could take elevators, and he could even fly. His necrotic kidney recovered, and he even stopped taking medication for that. This is how Dmitrii became Katerina's regular client. He usually came to her with health problems, when he wanted her to 'examine' (*prosmotret'*) the diagnoses made by numerous medical doctors in expensive clinics that he continued to visit. Sometimes she confirmed the diagnoses but monitored the medication regime, telling him what medicines to take and which to drop, out of the multitude prescribed by the doctors. (Katerina has a detailed knowledge of human anatomy, pathology and pharmaceuticals, and can easily converse with professional doctors in their own terms.) Sometimes she refuted the diagnosis and suggested her own version of what was wrong with him, sending him to undergo the appropriate tests. Most of the time, said Dmitrii, her verdicts were confirmed, and he continued to trust her.

Gradually, the two developed a relationship that was closer than that between client and magus. It involved more commitment, and was more ambivalent. Dmitrii always paid her for her treatment, but, in addition, he helped her a lot practically. He lent her money when needed, he found her apartments to rent when she was evicted, and once, early on, he invited her to join him for a quick trip to Finland: he was there on business, and he took her along, entirely at his expense, for her just to relax and to enjoy a change of air. This was a welcome break for Katerina, when it came up at one of my fieldwork stays. I asked her if they were 'getting it on', and she said no, not at all: he is actually afraid of women, that's why he is putting up with his strange wife, reduced to nothingness (*nikakaia*). After the trip, which she quite enjoyed, Katerina noted to me: 'You thought that he will court me – nothing of the kind! All those days he was talking only about his problems … This is how men see me – not as a woman, but as a *mag*. They are too scared of me to make passes, I am too strong for them. The only thing they want is to use my power to cover their back.'

The note of disenchantment that I thought I discerned in this remark was never explicitly confirmed by Katerina. She was a *mag*, not a woman, and this suited her well, and contributed to the charisma that she had constructed for herself. Also, Dmitrii was careful not to let her too deep inside his life, not even as a friend. He always discouraged her probing into the private spheres of his life on her own initiative. Neither did he ask her advice on business matters, until one time when he mentioned in passing that a couple of houses that he had built several months before were standing empty, that there were some buyers that were interested, but the deals had all gone wrong at the last moment. Katerina suggested working on the problem magically. Dmitrii had no confidence in this project, but Katerina said that she had a very strong spell, specifically for selling houses, that she wanted to test. She cast the spell over water in a bottle, which she took with her to the houses, where Dmitrii drove her one freezing winter night. She then sprinkled water inside the houses, first one and then the other. When Dmitrii turned up in her consulting room a couple of months later, again with some health problems that she did not think were at all significant, she asked him how it had gone with the houses. He answered casually that they had 'gone' (*ushly*) a long time ago. She was upset that it had not even occurred to him to thank her, and he said he had not connected this with magic: he had the interested buyers all along, they had just disappeared for some reason, and then came back. 'I didn't even care about these houses anyway', he said, 'My partners had already given me my share of the money for them, so I didn't give a damn.'

Katerina told me this story in her usual equanimous manner, without anger or explicit disappointment, but as a reason why she did not intend to work with him any more. 'If they think they can do it all by themselves, let them do it – why should I waste my time and power on them?', she remarked. Six months later, when we talked again, Dmitrii was still her client, calling on her every second month to confirm or refute another biomedical diagnosis.

These two cases give contexts in which spells can be used to remedy problems in all spheres of existence. Working life is only one of them, tightly intertwined with all the others. As I mentioned above, the use of spells is a sensitive matter; therefore, in discussing them here, I proceed, not from the subjectivities of specific clients, but from the spells as magical tools in their own right. In considering spells as 'icons of power', I give them the benefit of the doubt, taking at face value Katerina's conviction as regards their high potency. Spells are used because they work; if this is so, there must be some homology between the internal structure of the spells and the prevailing grids of power and patterns of subjectivity. To discern this homology, I shall analyse some spells from Katerina's collection. This analysis is guided by her comments and informed by her 'native exegesis' – as it happens, she has also given some thought to the question why spells might work.

Some examples of spells

Spell for a job interview
The following spell is recommended when you are going to a job interview. It is to be said three times just before leaving home. It has been modified to the recently adopted practice of sending your curriculum vitae CV when applying for a job; in this case you should say the spell three times on to the paper of the CV, 'so that it will absorb the energy of the spell'.

I am going to my lord; I am neither young nor old;
I am going to be hired; I am going to win the lord's heart.
He likes my face; he is not sick and tired of my soul.
Everybody will be surprised by my talents;
the lord will smile at my sweetness;
let him rejoice [*umiliat'sia*] at my words.
Should my master not send me – the baptized soul – packing.
My Lord Jesus Christ, our God, have mercy on us at every hour. Amen, Amen,
Amen.

'Lord' in this case is a translation of the archaic Russian word *barin*, the term which serfs (peasants who were the property of the landlord) used to refer to, or to address, their owner. Another word from the same semantic field, *khoziain*, owner or proprietor, here translated as 'master', conveys the same sense of one person being totally dependent on another, having his or her destiny left to the master's whim. Here, admission to a modern workplace (operating within the structures of the new market economy based on Western models) is conceived as hinging not on one's merits, not on one's competence or experience, but solely on the master's liking. This is not about the individual's right to be employed, nor does this order of things envisage any instance where one can appeal or protest. There are no social institutions that can support the person seeking to be hired in order to gain her livelihood. The only element that steers one's fate is the master's emotional disposition, his sheer liking, as unpredictable as the direction of the wind. Even before they are formalised, the working relationships are envisaged not as business-like transactions between a novice and a superior, whose power is relative and subject to other frames and limitations. Instead, it is an unlimited power of an absolute master that is at play here. One can not rely on the master's favourable disposition, nor can one rely on one's own merits speaking by themselves. But one can hope that the master's heart will somehow warm to the supplicant. It is not the rational appreciation of one's skills and professional potentials that will result in employment; instead, it is an endearment, enjoyment of the supplicant's personality, and smiles of complaisance. It is sheer emotional acceptance, totalised to embrace the whole person of the master's slave, by his face, soul and demeanour. The spell defines the supplicant as able-bodied and of an appropriate age for work (i.e. she has what it takes and can fit the right slot): if you are older, you have no chance of winning, no matter how qualified you are. The ego of the spell is abandoned to the mercy of the one with power, as completely as the human being, God's slave, is left at the mercy of God Himself. For this mercy one can only pray, and hope that it comes; never demand it, nor rely on one's right to grace. If this mercy is not forthcoming, one is kicked out, like a beggar or a dog, since it is to these categories that the colloquial Russian word *prognat'/vygnat'* (here translated as 'send packing') points back.

Spell against being laid off

Once one is employed at a workplace, there is no certainty about one's position. The next spell is used to prevent being laid off, which in Russia sometimes means being fired without prior notice, without any severance pay or any alternative job being offered – the actual situation is more aptly described by the verb 'to kick out/chuck out/send packing' – *vygnat/prognat'*.

A bottle of water is put in the foot of the bed where one sleeps. It is kept there for three days, and then carried to the workplace. At the workplace one washes one's face with the water, saying:

Here is where I have been, here is where I *shall* be.
Here is where I go, here is where I *shall* go. Amen.

In addition, one goes to the door of the boss's room, lifts one's right arm and says:

My right arm, my right leg, my right cause.
I have been, I am, I shall be.
In the name of the Father, the Son, and the Holy Spirit. Amen.

This spell takes on a much more assertive tone. Here, the ego is no longer a meek supplicant pleading for her master's liking. She is instead the fierce agent whose will and desire are shaped and directed by the words and the actions of the spell. The desired state here is that of continuity, where the subject strives to project the present to the future (conveyed by the juxtaposition of 'am' and 'shall be'). The aim is to perpetuate the ego's state of relative security, where one's work ensures one's survival tomorrow: the state of employment. There is a widespread understanding in Russia that water is one of the best agents to store the 'energy-information structures', a notion already familiar to the reader. As was mentioned before, *magi* routinely ask patients to procure bottles of water, to charge them with their energy that programmes desired changes. In the above spell, it is the energy of the ego's determination, accumulated in her over days, that grows stronger and is projected on to the water. Being objectified as water, it is then returned upon the body, splashed on to the face, the body's most visible part, the most crucial for the public representation of the self, but also the most vulnerable and the most inclined to betray whatever weakness the person harbours. The Russian saying has it that the best defence is attack; and for a person whose ancestors for generations were the master's serfs reduced to humble supplication, this form of defence needs a conscious step over one's state of intimidation: a feat of the transformation of consciousness, a mobilisation effort of all the resources of character.

Fashioned as it is, as a weapon of defence for the defenceless, this spell is conceived for confronting the powers-that-be. But it also draws the boundaries that can never be transcended, marked by the door of the boss's room. As in the rest of life, the war of the dispossessed is waged on their shared territory, while those with power have their retreat behind invisible doors. It is these thresholds, conjured in the spells of the popular subconscious, that work better than any armed guards to protect those who are invested with might. These are the ontologies of power, Bourdieu's invisible 'structuring structures' whose transgression cannot be engineered because they are encoded in all areas that form consciousness. These are the thresholds that are the last to crumble. It would seem that these boundaries can be removed when political and social systems disintegrate, in, for example, a revolution. But the texts of the spells suggest that these fault-lines of power and intimidation, these limits of agency, survive even such revolutions, as well as the other reforms of the much-touted concept of 'modernisation', leaving the fundamental ontologies of power intact. In the end it is the boss alone who decides whether or not the subordinate will have a chance of earning her living under his patronage. When it comes to firing an employee, it will ultimately be cast not as the formally respectful 'making redundant', but as 'kicking out' or 'getting rid of' (*vygnat'/prognat'*). In this situation the hired worker will have nothing but spells to resort to: no courts of appeal, no trade unions (the former do exist in today's Russia but are ensnared in bureaucracy and corruption; the latter vanished along with other Soviet institutions); not even muscle-men in leather jackets who stand for a semblance of civility and justice in the wilderness of the market beyond the salaried work sector. The Russian maxim, spelled out, like so many, in blunt language, sums it up nicely: 'I am the boss – you are shit; you are the boss – I am shit.'

Spells to protect against one's superiours

It can be imagined that one has not (as yet) happened to incur the wrath of one's principal master (in the case of *nachal'nik* [pl. *nacha'lniki*] it is wrath, *gnev*, not the undefined sign-less anger of the

185

dispossessed that is the emotion in question). This notwithstanding, there are still many actors at your workplace who can make your life thoroughly miserable. It can happen that a person has numerous bosses, big and small, and may find herself in a state of guerrilla war with a whole hierarchy of *nachal'niki*. It is well known in Russia that little *nachal'niki* are often meaner than bigger ones, never missing a chance to project on to subordinates the humiliations that they have been subjected to by their own superiors. *Pridirki*, picking on a person, finding faults with her, jumping at her without any reason, are so many small pinpricks that, accumulated, can add up to the magical *'negativy'* that can lead to *porcha*, ultimately destroying your body and your entire life. It is against these unmotivated outbreaks of nastiness on the part of superiors that the next spell is directed.

The master drives his carriage on, and whips his horses mercilessly.
Anger [*zlo*] boils within him, his gaze burns with wrath,
On their last breath, the horses drag their burden on.
The master always finds fault with them [*pridiraetsia*]:
Now they stand wrong, now they run wrong.
He lifts his arm and lashes out at the horses.
God, bless me.
You, God's slave [the name of the boss], stop jumping at me,
Stop tormenting me [*izgaliat'sia*]!
I wish by God that I could please God's slave (boss's name),
That he should not scold me thus without reason.
Holy Saints [*Ugodniki*], Holy Intercessors, Holy martyrs! Be my protection!
Hallowed be Thy name, oh Lord the Father, the Son, and the Holy Spirit, amen.

Katerina pointed out to me that spells, as finished products of poetic expression, are structured according to a set pattern. First, the stage is set, the situation is evoked that describes, and conveys, the tone-feeling (Peircian First) of the state in which the user of the spell suffers. In my terms, this part of the spell can be seen as the semiotic Object of her emotional state. These introductory, evocative brush-strokes are the Icons of the individual's predicament, because they contain the same emotion that consumes the victim and forcefully communicate it to the world. This emotion may not be named: it can lack Representamen, being even more psychologically unsettling and physically destructive for that.

In the above spell, the ego identifies herself with the horses dragging a carriage driven by a raging master. This identification of the employee with the carriage-dragging horses tells us more about the subjectivity of the spell-user than any amount of description (which, presented by an informant in an interview or in an informal conversation, might well be seen by a Western observer as belonging to the 'lamentation' genre [or *plach*], in the self-victimising spirit of the stereotyped Russian 'slave soul', as some American social psychologists would have it cf. Rancour–Laferriere 1995). Instead of general lamentations on the hardships of life, the poetics of the spell conveys the enslavement, the labour that is felt as more than human. It evokes the strain to please the one who holds the reigns, the impossibility of doing so no matter how great the effort deployed, and the pain of arbitrary punishment when the whiplash lands on the horses' backs at the whim of the rider.

The spell becomes a strikingly expressive Representamen for a complex of unspeakable emotions. These emotions are impossible to describe in so many words, but they are easily recognisable for those who share their Ground – the life-world in which the spell is used. Faithfully serving animals at peace with their task of dragging the carriage become panic-driven beasts when the lash stings their backs no matter what they do, no matter whether they stand still or career madly onwards. What boils in the *barin* (the *nachal'nik* of bygone times) is denoted in the spell by the Russian word *zlo*, the word that has already been encountered on these pages in the conversation between the *mag* Tatiana and the mother of the boy afflicted by *porcha* (Chapter 3). In that case, Tatiana appealed to the woman not to hold *zlo* against the failed in-laws of her son. The first dictionary gloss of the word '*zlo*' is 'evil', while in common speech it is often translated as 'grudge', bad feelings, and serves well as a Representamen for anger. But what burns in the barin's gaze is '*gnev*', wrath, establishing firmly the power-hierarchy of the protagonists, the 'force' or 'might structures' (as in the Russian term '*silovye*' or '*vlastnyie struktury*'). These structures of might underlie all other relations, and the spell does not challenge them. The horses are there to draw the carriage; this is in their nature to do so, and this configuration is sealed by the spell, iconically conveyed by it as one of life's givens. What is contested, and what is targeted as an object of change through the spell, is the *barin's* evil way of handling the faithful horses.

The way the *barin* treats his horses, and, by implication, the way the hypothetical user of the spell perceives she is treated by her superiors, is defined by the Russian word *izdevat'sia* (the spell uses its stronger and more colloquial and archaic synonym *'izgaliat'sia'*), yet another widely used Russian term impossible to translate directly into English. *Izdevat'sia* means to make a mockery, or a travesty, of a person in a singularly cruel way; it could be compared with 'ganging', except that *'izdevat'sia'* is used more often than not in a one-to-one, face-to-face interpersonal context. It means to torment or humiliate in a painful way, making fun of one's weaknesses, taking gleeful pleasure in the victim's suffering. This verb, denoting despicable harassment, inflicted by a stronger party on the weaker or defenceless one, also implies a hierarchy of power between the subject and the agent of *izdevatel'stvo*. It must be noted, however, that this very strong word has now to some extent become diluted in colloquial parlance. Thus, in friendly pique when one party is making fun of another's weak points, the latter might well retort in mild reproach: 'are you *izdevaesh'sia*?' This can be compared with the common use of the word 'betrayal' (*predatel'stvo*), whose potency is likewise diluted by overuse. In the above spell, however, the word carries its full charge denoting deprivation, by its being placed in an appropriate context and by using its stronger, more archaic variant.

The second part of the spell, Katerina told me, contains the exposition of the desired state of affairs, as straightforward request (do this and that), or through presenting the wished-for picture. In addition, this spell, in its middle part, portrays the vision of the good life, as desired by the individual in question. It is not that the horses have toppled their rider and maybe trampled him to death. The horses' natural state of being is to drag the carriage, and this state is not contested, but rather confirmed by the spell. In this ideal world, the configuration of power remains unchanged, and the horses still charge forward with their *barin*. What is changed is the *barin*'s disposition: he has stopped harassing the horses with his lash, whipping them in a needlessly cruel way. In this vision of the desirable state of affairs, instead of the forceful word *'izdevatel'stvo'* the *barin* reproaches or chastises his subordinate; what the ego of the spell wants is that these reprimands should not come 'without reason'. The *barin* should drop his 'evil', taking a liking in his horses instead; they should become 'pleasing' for him.

It is the final part of the spell that carries the agentive thrust of this magical bullet, evoking the presence of those forces of the cultural imaginary who are sought out to use their supernatural powers to bring about the desired situation. The strength of the spell, Katerina told me, is directly connected with the place of these invoked beings in the cosmological hierarchy of powers. In this case, the persons summoned are saints of the Russian Orthodox Church, addressed at large, as a community, rather than called individually by names. They are those who stand before God, those who are dear or pleasing to Him, as the spell's ego, God's slave, should be pleasing to his *barin* (*ugodniki* comes from the archaic word '*ugodnyi*', pleasing or endearing). They are Intercessors, *Zastupniki*, from the verb '*zastupat'sia*', those who defend people, represent their interests before the higher powers, supplicate for them to the mighty, and mediate between these slaves of God and God Himself in case of His wrath. And there are Holy martyrs, who know what the suffering of the whipped horses, of arbitrary pain and humiliation, is.

Spell to obtain favour from one's superiours

The next spell is used in order to obtain favours from superiors. The word used in the title of this spell is '*milost*'. *Milost*' is an archaic word most directly glossed as God's grace, as in the set expression '*milost*' *Bozhia*'. In this combination, *milost*' is the favourable attitude of God that results in the ego being specially endowed with, for example, talent or luck beyond average. *Milost*' was also used in pre-revolutionary times in peasants' dealings with landlords. It was associated with the good disposition of a monarch or any other authoritarian ruler, as unpredictable as God's grace, that resulted in the ego's swift promotion or high reward. *Milost*' is granted you by someone whose power over you is limitless, on whom you are in a situation of total dependency, and whose benevolence towards you will open totally new horizons in terms of your ability to improve your life. As God's grace, *milost*' belongs to the category of minor miracles, to hope for, to pray for, but never to rely on, much less to demand as your right. According to this logic, the spell is used to manipulate the agency of higher powers, to secure the desired state of affairs which is impossible to obtain by any other means.

I, the slave of God, shall venture forth, into God's world,
There is no one who will cross my path on the broad street,
There is no one who either crosses it or blocks it,
There is no one who would say 'no' to me, God's slave.

There is no one who would distract me with their speeches,
There is no one who would convince me against my will.
God's light will illuminate me,
His holy icon will bless me,
A cloud in the sky will shroud me over,
A multitude of stars will pour over me.
Just as the new moon cannot be thrown out of the sky,
So I cannot be thrown out/interrupted in my work/cause/plan.
Nobody can break me.
For centuries I shall stick to my guns,
Not letting go of my work/cause/plan.
Everything will happen the way I wish it.
In the name of the Son, the Father, and the Holy Spirit. Amen. Amen. Amen.

This spell is amongst Katerina's favourites: she says that this is a very strong one that really works. It is used for people who are indecisive and weak, are easily distracted from their purpose, persuaded to do things against their will. It is a spell for those who are vacillating in their standpoint, who have difficulties in bringing their projects to fruition, or in carrying their work to a glorious end. In my terms, this spell serves to reinforce the ego's intentionality, to strengthen one's will to make it possible to confront other competing wills, designs and agendas. An intriguing question that this comment poses is the tension between the constructed goal of the spell, the self's agency that needs strengthening, and the choice of words in its title, which transfers the source of agency from the self to higher powers, whether the heavenly God's grace, or the earthly, like the grace of *nachal'stvo*.

The firmness of nature's laws, the inexorable movement of celestial bodies is through this spell projected on to the life of the ego, endowing her presence at the workplace with unquestioned, solid quality. The ego's existence in her working context will be as impossible to alter as it is impossible to move the moon from the heavenly sphere. The spell talks about the work to be accomplished, the cause to be fulfilled, the plan to be brought to fruition (all possible translations of the noun '*delo*'). What is at stake in situations which this spell invokes is that the individual's only desire is to be given a conducive environment to accomplish what she deems crucial in her working life. It is this configuration that, in some situations, is conceived as a minor miracle, only achievable through the grace or favourable disposition of the powers that be.

Spells against being eased out from one's workplace

Thrown on the mercy of powers not of one's own making, and being enmeshed in the configurations of forces over which one has no legal, social, or other rational levers, one can experience various emotions. The ego's subjectivity in these situations of total powerlessness varies across the entire range, from rage and revolt, possibly involving the spilling of blood, against these powers, to all kinds of perfectly conscious efforts to adapt, please and accommodate, by whatever means, in the attempt to win sympathy and favour or to acquire a liking on the part of one's environment by co-opting supernatural powers to secure grace or *milost'*. Or this same subjectivity can plunge to the nadir of despair before the individual's total inability to prevent the encroachment of the world on the self, to relieve the continued pressure, the 'pecking away' at the self, just as a vulture pecks at its prey, until total extinction. Here we encounter the longing to become invisible, to fade away, a desire all too familiar to us from childhood, for example, when we are subject to adults' anger or when we are the victims of bullying. This desire can take various forms; its extreme form may even be to turn into something utterly repellent to all, particularly one's assailants, even to oneself. This form of subjectivity is one of unspeakable abjection, beyond mere words. It is encapsulated in a spell, as follows:

The user should come to her workplace before everybody else, go to the toilet, and say:

As people do not eat shit in an out-house,
So my bosses should stop eating me;
As people sit in the out-house,
So I should sit at my workplace.
As people cannot do without an out-house,
So God's slave [boss's name] will not be able to do without me.
Key, lock, tongue. Amen.

The emotional thrust of this spell is built on the potency of the images of abjection juxtaposed with the everyday and infused with the intrinsic existential craving to protect the self, to make it inviolable, secure and prosperous. The spell conveys the subjectivity of the individual cornered by life. It tells how miserable life can become when the favour of the boss is not forthcoming. The process of evacuation of bodily waste is difficult to interrupt once it is under way, and this quality of continuity is conferred on the professional persona. It iconically presents the ego as irreplaceable for the functioning of the social unit, and for the boss's continued entitlement – as Katerina commented to me, what is more necessary than the toilet in city premises? The need for the self is conveyed through the impossibility of the other's existence without her, no matter what one thinks of the ego's qualities. In contrast to other spells, in this one no celestial, natural forces, nor any of the Orthodox social imaginary are summoned to consolidate its impact. There is only language, the uttering of the words, that under lock and key will forever remain concealed from the prying and evil influence of others. The extremity and the liminality of such a situation, when one is driven to the point of identifying with faeces as the only way to fight back evokes in itself a survival potential comparable to that offered by the intercession of saints and archangels.

Spell against being 'eased out' of life

The title of the next spell could be rendered approximately as 'When they try to wipe you from the face of the earth'. The Russian original *'Esli vas szhivaiut so sveta belogo'* invokes the situation when one is slowly and painfully shut off from the whole wide world in an inconspicuous but singularly painful way. *'Szhivat'* is a derivative from the verb *'zhit'*, to live. There are two verbs with this root that connote gradual retreat from life, the stealthy approach of 'non-life', contrived through someone's care. One can be squeezed out of the living space of one's apartment or one's workplace, by one's mother-in-law, neighbours, a spouse, or by one's boss, as in the verb *'vyzhivat iz ...'*. It is long and meticulous process, something that does not happen overnight, but through deliberate effort of another, doing the same work as a drop of water that erodes stone (as in the Russian proverb 'Water can wear down e'en stone itself'). The end goal of this adverse agency, in the case of *vyzhivat'*, is to deprive someone of living space, of her livelihood and security; as a result, although one might find oneself out in the cold, one might still hope to survive. In a related verb, *szhivat' so sveta*, one is, as it were, squeezed or edged out, not only of one's dwelling place, but of life itself. The perfective form of this verb, *szhit' so sveta*, means to destroy or completely annihilate. When a person feels her situation is of this character (or when a *mag* considers it to be such), when there are no other defences to resort to, then the following spell is in order:

To be read on the waning of the moon, at sunset, just before dusk, twelve days in a row:

There are twelve knives, guarded by thirteen watchmen, twelve saints and Judas.
I shall approach those steel knives, I shall bow low to the watchmen [*poklonius' do zemli*], I shall talk to them in a pleasant voice, I shall plead:
Judas, look at me!
Let people no longer fear and despise me!
Let me no longer be persecuted by people for hundred years!
You have been hurt and despised by everyone [*obizhali*, past tense verb from the noun *obida*],
You have been kicked out of everywhere;
You have been spat upon, you have been cursed.
Take upon yourself my sorrows, too.
Take upon yourself the twelve knives and the thirteen watchmen.
Word, tongue, lock, the threshold of the church. Amen.

This spell conveys the raw quality of feeling, felt before it is expressed, and maybe too painful to be spelled in the agent's own words. It is the choice of the intercessor that communicates this First in its visceral existential quality. It does it more effectively than many words that could be used to describe the indescribable – the subjectivity of humiliation, suffering, deprivation and loneliness at the extreme limits of human abjection. The figure to whom the self of the spell supplicates is not the suffering Christ, but the figure who is unique in the Christian imaginary by virtue of the hatred that has been heaped on him for centuries, of the isolation of this personage over all other humans, beyond redemption, beyond any flicker of hope.

The deep mystery of Judas that titillated the imagination of many interpreters over the centuries is his irreplaceability in the Christian plan for the redemption of humanity. As Katerina mused, commenting on this spell, Christ could die without the interference of Judas; but Judas's betrayal adds another dimension to Christ's suffering, and Christ's sacrifice is therefore also that of Judas. Resurrection and worship, however, are reserved by myth to Christ alone. In Katerina's words, if someone knew what it meant to end up in the grip of Karma, it was Judas. He was the one who knew how it was to become a victim of circumstances, where the one who is spat upon cannot even deny his prosecutors the justice of their abusive actions; how it was to be the one who, by the force of destiny, was removed beyond the confines of minimally shared morality space. The semiotic First of this spell is the depth of despair of a person cut off from all hope: from any possibility of resorting to help or consolation, not even the consolation of the thought that one's position is righteous or morally justified. This is the ultimate loneliness of the unwitting perpetrator of the crime which is none of his doing, for whom all the normally available reserves of compassion have dried up. This is the last horror of the situation of severance, not only of social ties, but of the mere possibility of these ties, the self's deprivation of entitlement to the most basic expressions of humanness. The supplicant singles out Judas as her last redeemer, thus placing herself not among human kind as a whole but among its most disaffected, jettisoned as ultimate refuse. The last hope of the one upon whom everybody else spits is that she will be helped by he who has forsaken all hope. Judas is therefore the only one who may agree to take on the sorrows of the supplicant, leaving her the one last glimpse of hope – the hope that the burden of the world's enmity will be lifted, even if only a little.

Spells to use in business

Not all the spells tap the primordial depth of existential conundrums. Some of them are concise and pragmatic. According to Katerina, spells do not solve deeper problems of relational configurations, psychological disturbances, fatal flaws of character or trials of fate. Rather, spells are light and precise weapons that address problems situationally and temporarily, giving the user a short respite to gather her forces for longer and more arduous battles. Spells are used abundantly in trade and in small business, such as the following ones:

To read over the object to be sold, making the sign of the cross over it:

I am the merchant, I am always brilliant/successful/excellent in my trade (*vsegda molodets*)
My goods will be sold to you. Money to money. Our money to us, your goods to you. Amen.

✤ ✤ ✤

To read on the honey with which to smear yourself before you go to the place of the trade:

As bees swarm, so all the merchants will come to me, the merchant. Let them praise my merchandise, so that they will snatch it from my hands.
Let my chests and treasure-trove overflow with wealth. Amen.

Bread is baked on the waxing of the moon. This spell is read over the dough before baking:

As you, dough, will rise and grow bigger, so I shall grow in my status, in my fame and in my wealth. Amen.

The first earnings from the sale of the merchandise are put at the four corners of the table. Three candles are lit on the table. Stamp, clap and read:

Altyn Khatan has come here, he has taken my goods. One has bought, another has saved [the money]. Let me also have all and everything. Amen.

As Katerina told me, one of the most important skills of the magus working with spells is to choose the right one that best suits the client's predicament in terms of its 'energy frequencies' or 'energo-information patterns'. The way I read it in terms of this study is that, from the narrative of the client and from her entire gestalt, the magus must discern, and give an appropriate form to, the unspeakable, the Peircian First of the problematic situation in which the client finds herself. In Peircian phenomenology, Firstness is feeling before thought, a quality of immediate consciousness prior to objectification or cognition. In the kaleidoscope of everyday occurrences and incidents, the Seconds of the individual's life, 'encounters with hard fact, the undeniable shock of contact with … the sensuous, reluctant world' (1932: 1.307) – may change in rapid succession from bad to worse. Reason and volition fall apart, and what remains is only the First of inescapable abjection. It is this First that the magus should discern and try to remedy. As in the case of terms of affliction, the first step is to capture this diffuse experience in a manageable form. Spells are poetic units for comparable Firsts, distilled by culture over centuries; they are what Susanne Langer calls 'significant forms'.

Langer develops her notion of significant forms in connection with nonverbal arts – music and dance – but it is readily applicable to spells as well. She defines significant form as 'an articulate expression of feeling, reflecting the verbally ineffable and therefore unknown form of sentience' (Langer 1953: 39). Its vital import is something actual that is revealed, articulated or made manifest. It is 'a virtual object, like a rainbow or a shadow', that conveys, or 'gives a clear connection to', the reality found in the world. Poetic presentation, rather than representation, of the First, the spell sets forth 'the pure quality, or semblance ...., apart from familiar worldly attributes and relations' (ibid.: 49–50). By virtue of its dynamic structure, these poetic units express the forms of vital experience that the everyday discursive forms of language are unable to convey. It is an articulate form having import without a conventional reference, presenting to conscious awareness something that was beyond it, 'feeling, life, motion and emotion' (ibid.), in the words of Langer. The factor of significance in it is not logically discriminated; it is felt as a quality rather than recognised as a function. Conveying these patterns of sentience, spells become their instant Representamina, complex signs in the clients' consciousness. But they are signs different from conventional linguistic ones, acting more as nonverbal significate forms than as verbal discursive units: herein lies their 'strangeness' and 'otherness', their magicality. They become Representamina that 'have significate effect' rather than 'stand for'. They are forms immediately given to perception, and yet reaching beyond themselves, 'a semblance charged with reality' (Langer 1953: 52). They mean indexically, not only or primarily by producing 'another sign in the mind of the Interpreter', but affecting the Interperter's sentience and practice.

The emotional and pragmatic import of spells, as in the case of other artistic forms considered by Langer, consists in the fact that they present, instead of represent or suggest as conventional language does, the nondiscursive content of feeling. As other tools of magic described before, spells act indexically because they present iconically the homologous Firsts, the structures of immediate feeling. But this similarity of the Firsts stems from another, deeper, form of iconicity – the similarities in the structures of coercive power and in the subjectivities of subordination and dependency, helplessness and humiliation, acceptance and rebellion that have remained unchanged throughout each and every tumultuous political and economic transformation. Like other magical tools, spells are designed to change the situation through the seemingly naïve indexicality of Copy and Contact (and it should be recalled that it is only the short-term situation that spells are designed to change). The logic of their action is encoded in their tripartite structure, akin, as it were, to a stage missile: the present state, the desired state, and the forces that are called upon to effect the transformation. These stages work semiotically, through giving Seconds to Firsts, or Representamina to Objects. Inasmuch as they are significant forms, spells work indexically, by producing significate effects, in subjectivity, behaviour, and thus in intersubjectivity, sociality and environment. Spells are designed to actualise changes, and it is no wonder that they have been used for centuries to exactly this effect. As other icons used in the world of Russian magic, spells are, in their own ways, the icons of power. Like other icons described on these pages, they are constructed as such through the shared Thirds, habits of interpretation that persisted through centuries (and here is a subtle difference between the notion of habitus and the Third: habitus varies across social groups, and is subject to dramatic changes in time; while the habits of interpretation, the Thirds, pertain to deeper cultural structures, ontologies of power, that die hardest and modify the most alien, and most 'modern', imported institutions).

Notes

1. Spells appear to have been at their most popular in Russia in the seventeenth century, when most records of magic were first made systematically. Some of the spells are indistinguishable from Orthodox prayers, and others have references to pre-Christian times and pagan mythology. Russian spells have much in common with those found in the folklore of other cultures, e.g. Scandinavian, Anglo-Saxon, Balkan Slav and Greek. See Ryan (1999), who has a section on spells in the history of Russian magic.

2. V.I. Kharitonova compares spells used in Russian village folk magic with chants and incantations used by Siberian shamans, and both of these to music therapy. She writes: 'The fabric of the voice [of the practitioner] plus repetition of certain intonational and melodical units act in the same way as music does' (Kharitonova 1995: 78). She develops this thought in another work, saying that 'in altered states of consciousness, ... the known texts of *kamlanie* [shamanic séances that include chants], the rhythms of the drum, ... as well as the texts of spells and incantations, intensify the non-ordinary

mode of brain activities in the people who are disposed accordingly' (Kharitonova 1999: 48)

3. Malinowski, in analysing Trobriand magic spells, coined the term 'verbal missiles', to convey the efficacy of magical words. See Tambiah (1990: 73–76).

4. The components of Trobriand spells singled out by Malinowski were: phonetic effects, including onomatopoeic words; imperatives that evoked, stated and commanded certain feeling states and certain consequences; and constructions that retrospectively referred back to myths of origins and the pedigree of ancestors. Thus, he recognised the connection of magic and emotion, reference to tradition as legitimation, and its pragmatic character as instrumental rather than expressive action (Tambiah 1990).

5. Malinowski spoke about the 'coefficient of weirdness' that magic speech in the Trobriands contained as compared with the higher 'coefficient of intelligibility' of ordinary speech. This was indexed by strange and archaic grammatical forms, words containing esoteric meanings, and strange mythological and metaphoric references. (Tambiah 1999).

Chapter 7
The Magic of Business and the Fostering of Hope

The central theme of this book has been to show how magical practices can work to augment individual human agency in a society where the formal channels of agency are limited, and to change subjectivity, for example, by attenuating and modifying psychologically destructive and socially disruptive emotions. In this chapter, I shall develop further the view of magic as an aspect of the existential safety net operating in conditions of 'precarious presence' (see Rodriguez Larreta 2002). In the 'jungle' of the brave new Russia, magic can be seen as a way of lending *illusio* to those playing tough social games more akin to Russian roulette. It can serve to offer the lost sense of tomorrow, a tool for fostering hope. In the previous chapters, I have shown how magic helps people manage diverse spheres of their life, where health, love, family and business are tied up in inseparable knots. In this final chapter, I shall take a closer look at the spheres of business, commerce and employment, and at the ways in which magic is used in these domains. I shall try to show that, in conditions where trust has disappeared, magic can be used as a psychosocial mechanism comparable to the strategies of trust-formation, but giving something different – faith rather than trust; and that it can work as a tool to give the existence of precarious presence a temporal dimension and a subjective feeling of control. Both of these are necessary if the 'fields of social games' are to exist at all in the absence of any clearly outlined and conscientiously adhered-to rules of the game.

This chapter is based on the story of the struggle of one individual, a young man whom I shall call Misha, whose unsatisfying visit to the Centaur centre was described in Chapter 1. Misha's story is worth relating in greater detail, because it provides a cross-section of Russian life through a period of time, offering insight into several social domains, including the market and business relations. These relations did not appear after perestroika out of the blue. In the command economy of Soviet times, citizens purchased goods available through the networks of state distribution, where supply was regulated by arbitrary 'planning' mechanisms rather than by demand (see Verdery 1996; Nagengast 1991, among many others). If 'market' is defined as 'commercial activity to effect the exchange of commodities' (Webster), then 'market' undoubtedly thrived in the nooks and crannies of the Soviet structures. One of its forms was barter, being the most direct way through which the exchange of commodities was effected. Barter was, and remains, an important type of transaction in Soviet and post-Soviet times (see, e.g. Ledeneva 1998; Seabright 2000; Chornyi 2000; Humphrey 2002b, Ch. 2). The so-called 'black market' worked using market mechanisms and provided certain sectors of society with quality clothes, music recordings, books, theatre tickets, and other scarce goods in high demand (*defitsit*).

However, this market of sorts operated outside state structures, was criminalised, and furthermore was considered by many as thoroughly immoral. As part of his initial perestroika reforms, Gorbachev made an attempt to decriminalise a small fraction of this 'market' by allowing 'cooperatives'. These initiated post-Soviet commerce and the 'support infrastructure' around it, the criminal and para-criminal protection business known as *krysha*, 'roof' (see the collection by Ledeneva and Kurkchiyan 2000, especially chapters by Volkov and by Galeotti, and also Humphrey 2002b Ch. 5). When market relations were legalised after perestroika, it was those with the old social capital who became the new actors on the market. They came partly from the leading ranks of industry, and partly from those who had previously operated the 'black market', and who were competent in commercial activity, and enjoyed access to material and social resources.

Misha's story

Misha belonged to none of these. He had to do it all by himself, starting from scratch. Misha was born in a small town in Siberia. His father died when Misha was very young; his mother was a doctor, working hard to make ends meet. The two children were brought up by their grandmother, a despotic woman with a heavy hand and an iron will. Grandmother saw to it that the two brothers were baptised. Misha was ten years old at the time, a young pioneer. His baptism was arranged in secret from Misha's mother, who was an atheist and a communist, and would never have allowed it; so, the grandmother lied to her daughter that she had taken the children to see her relatives three hundred kilometres away, which at the time was the nearest place with a working church. Misha's memories of his baptism were undramatic: 'Just lots of screaming kids dragged to be baptised'. Afterwards he was grateful to his grandmother, and came to see this baptism as at least a form of protection, one he later came to need badly.

Misha graduated from a small engineering college in the neighbouring city, and started to work as a builder on a construction site. He was a hard worker, with a pleasant personality, plenty of energy, and with organisational abilities, and he did well. He spent his first savings on going to a resort on the Black Sea, where he met his wife to be, a woman from Moscow. A couple of months later he took time off, went to Moscow, married his wife, and settled down in her apartment, where he got registered, thus obtaining the much-coveted Moscow *propiska*.

This was the beginning of the 1980s, the time of 'stagnation'. This notwithstanding, Misha found many possibilities to further his career. He worked on construction sites, starting from the lowliest menial jobs, and in a couple of years he was promoted to become a foreman (*prorab*). Realising that his degree from the small Siberian college did not give him any credentials in the capital, he started evening courses in a Moscow construction college.

He plugged into the social networks of his wife, which, together with his own perseverance, brought him a good position at the 'Ministry of Bread Products', a peculiar establishment of Soviet times in charge of the distribution of 'bread products' (*khleboprodukty*) over the whole country. It consisted of the departments that were responsible for sending the quotas of bread products to the factories grouped according to the various branches of industry. One department of the bread products industry distributed bread orders to the factories of the chemical industry of the Russian Federation, another supplied the oil industries, a third the timber industries. The factories that baked bread received orders to send their production to the factories of the petrochemical industries, and the representatives of these industries would come to the Bread Ministry to obtain better quotas from their respective departments. Misha was put in charge of one such department, and he created an entire network of contacts with middle-range industrial bosses over the whole country[1]. He was happy about this job, one that involved a lot of human contact and travelling all over the Soviet Union; and he had good prospects of being promoted within the Ministry, when perestroika started.

The Bread Ministry was promptly closed down, and its numerous employees found themselves on the street. Misha was among them. That was a situation hardly conducive to family harmony, because his wife was adamant that 'the man of the household should earn his share'. The new market opened up new possibilities for business, and Misha plunged headlong into this new element. One of his projects was selling fake Adidas sports shoes, produced by a small cooperative in Leningrad and transported directly to the people at the factories of those industries he had got to know during his time at the Bread Ministry. This was a time that Misha recalled with a certain nostalgia: the goods were sold in the security of the factory gymnasia, behind closed doors and safeguarded by agreements with factory reps whom Misha knew personally. There were no racketeers, and no 'roof' was needed; nobody hunted him down with a gun asking for a share of his earnings. But both the cooperative in Leningrad and the factories whose workers bought their produce were closed down, and the business stopped.

Misha started many more projects, both in commerce and in the construction business; but nothing really succeeded. He started to wonder. 'I was a young man, full of energy and the desire to work, to "spin" [*krutit'sia*, see Pesmen 2000] and to make money. People liked me and were eager to deal with me; yet still, nothing really ever worked out. There was nothing wrong with me intrinsically; so, it must have been something else. The trouble was that I didn't understand what that something else was.'

His wife introduced Misha to an important man. She called this man by his first name, something that indicated a special relationship between the two, a relationship into whose nature Misha preferred not to inquire. Nobody ever mentioned this man's surname; everybody called him Godfather. Godfather was a short, stocky man with a muscular body and closely cropped hair. Misha sensed that he had enormous power. He had no official post, he did not belong to any business company or state institution, and Misha knew nothing either of his origins or his past. The only thing he did know was that Godfather had contacts on all levels of society, and that he was a brilliant fixer in many areas, including that of residential construction, a booming business in Moscow in the middle of the 1990s. One of Godfather's many roles was to mediate between major municipal customers and small, private, temporary teams that carried out construction work. Municipal customers paid big money, of which only a fraction went to the builders themselves, but when Godfather oversaw the work, the foreman did not have to worry about bureaucratic red tape, supply of building materials, or harassment by authorities. Godfather took care of everything, and the builders' teams only had to worry about the manual labour, which Godfather demanded be done with speed and quality.

Godfather offered Misha the job of organising a project for the reconstruction of a monastery a couple of hundred kilometres from Moscow. Big money was promised, and Misha put together a group of builders who operated more like a military unit. They lived in the monastery, they ate the frugal food together with the monks, they were not allowed to leave the site during the several months in which the work was planned to be done, and there was a complete prohibition on alcohol amongst the workers. This was an unusual arrangement, but the people concerned agreed to it because big money was promised. Even Misha himself did not get any advance payment, awaiting instead deferred gratification the same way as his subordinates did.

The work was going fast by Russian standards, when, after three months, Godfather himself arrived at the site. Among other things, he inspected the ledgers, of which Misha was in charge, and questioned the way the business was done. Misha was hurt (*obidelsia*, was hit by *obida*, as he told me). 'If he didn't trust me I might as well have left', he explained. Misha left the site in anger (or, rather, in *obida*), without receiving any money for the slave labour he had been doing for the last six months. What was worse, he parted with Godfather on bad terms, and Godfather's enemies were known not to live long.

Misha was gripped by extreme anxiety, and the violent anger with which his wife met him did not make matters any easier. 'You idiot, if you could not make use of such a contact, then you are a useless parasite,' she screamed at him, 'You'd better find yourself something else to do to bring some money home, otherwise I'll throw you out'. Full of *obida*, Misha walked out. He had neither money nor a place to live. The only thing he did have was a dilapidated old car (described in Chapter 1) that became his only means of survival, as an unauthorised taxi cab (there are hundreds of such private cars roaming the streets of Moscow, ready to offer a lift several times cheaper that the registered taxis, at any hour of the day). That was when his health started to give way: he suddenly felt that his body was falling apart. He was plagued with back pains, and his stomach ached. The doctors diagnosed an ulcer and prescribed a strict diet, which he could not even dream of keeping because he had no kitchen in which to cook.

He found shelter with his former business partners, a group of traders from India operating in Moscow. They were men of his age (in their early thirties), who worked in the business which had started up in Moscow in the early 1980s, then operating as a black market, and acquiring semi-legal status after perestroika. They shipped clothes, fabrics, teas and spices from India, and sold the goods at the big markets that proliferated in Moscow by that time. Over the years the Indians had developed their protection and problem-solving networks, and their business was doing well. They allowed Misha to stay in their apartment, sharing it with four other men, for a token price that he would pay back when his affairs improved. Living from hand to mouth, he would drive his car around, as he desperately looked for something more substantial to hang on to.

That was when my mother met him, flagging him down in the street for a lift. He was polite and extremely reliable, and a calm and inoffensive driver (a rare and precious quality in Moscow) and my mother became one of his permanent clients. I got to know Misha through my mother, admired his driver's skills, and myself started to call him for a lift. As we rode along, we talked, and he became an important informant on questions of Russian life in general and commerce and business in particular. We never became friends in any accepted meaning of the word; he always carefully kept his distance, and I never managed to persuade him to address me in the second person singular, by '*ty*', a sign of informality and familiarity in Russia. But he was always ready to talk, and to help in many other ways. He was one of the very few people who readily agreed to be taped, in order to 'lend scholarship a helping hand'.

His life was not lacking in business opportunities. He actively looked for jobs, and actually found some, in construction work and renovating houses, as well as in various business deals that involved buying and selling. But he had no luck: over and over again business transactions ended, not only in his being swindled, but in dramatic and humiliating put-downs.

The ethos of contract, the cornerstone of business in the West, is by no means unknown to Russian entrepreneurs. In the West, trust between individuals, and in legal institutions, is important in terms of respecting a contract; yet no less significant are moral and legal sanctions against the breach of contract. Such sanctions are absent in Russian business life; the body of requisite law is still being drawn up. Even if some rules and regulations do exist, the members of law-enforcement agencies in situ are human beings employed by the State, and to survive, they have to supplement their meagre salaries with private contributions from interested parties.

My informants say that now, as I write this, the situation is better than it was in 1999, when Misha's life hit rock bottom, as did the lives of many others after the shock of the *'defolt'* of 1998. Now, in 2003, they say, the pie is already divided, the various spheres of influence are distributed, and there are almost no spectacular killings in broad daylight any more.

Even if now there are more and clearer rules in 'market economy' (and in dealings that are involved, in Russia generally glossed as *'biznes'*), they are still formulated vaguely and enforced selectively; you can always influence those responsible for law enforcement if you have connections and, most importantly, money (the two go hand-in-hand); and also, if you forge human bonds with specific individuals who can decide your fate here and now. And the creation of human bonds is always a possibility: Dale Pesmen got to the root of the issue when she noted, quoting her informant, that 'everybody wants something, but only through somebody' (2000).

Impersonal contacts in the public sphere can often be transformed into personal contacts based on give-and-take, more akin to the Soviet-type *blat* (but, as Ledeneva [1998] argues, different from it in many important aspects). Money and gifts are essential elements in this interaction, but they are not always all there is to it. To give a bribe in Russia is an exquisite social art; if you do it wrong, you can land yourself in worse trouble. Bribery and other forms of corruption at the high levels of business are one of the areas left that still hinge on personal connections: it is here that an intermediary is needed, to direct the money to the right person, and to arrange a situation of bribe-giving that would be relatively safe for those involved; or, sometimes, to act as an intermediary himself (ibid.). Where formal (business or bureaucratic) contacts are personalised, personal qualities of the actors come to the fore. Money, prestige and presents are all social factors that should not be overlooked, but they are nothing short of useless unless the individual possesses personal power of persuasiveness, charm and attraction. In the previous chapters I wrote about the 'cultural designs' that work, as it were, like keys, to open the hearts of the healers' clients. But these keys, to a degree, must be involved in all other human interactions as well: formal transactions in Russia are personalised to a much greater degree than one is accustomed to in the West. Therefore, one's success in business tends to hinge, apart from one's formal merits and competence, on that quality of human personality that allows people, to use the famous words of Dale Carnegie (translated, well-loved and much quoted in Russia) 'to make friends and influence people.'

Carnegie's coupling of friendship and influence, which suggests that friendship ties are there as a kind of lever for manipulating people for one's personal needs, might have rung false in Soviet times. Friendship was then, indeed, a variety of love, a social institution that was highly emotionally charged, even as it was indispensable for people's everyday survival. In her analysis of *blat*, Ledeneva (1998) stresses the fact that, in Soviet-time friendship, the affective component was tightly intertwined with the instrumental one, and that people had high moral stakes in downplaying this instrumental component. Indeed, she singles this out as one of the strategies of 'misrecognition' that allowed *blat* to exist in the first place. She also discusses deep changes in the institution of friendship that post-Soviet social and economic transformations entailed. Among them are growing separation between friendship and business, and a general decrease in the significance of friendship for people's lives. This notwithstanding, there is also an opposite tendency of personalizing formal relationships, as Ledeneva also notes. This being so, and in the absence of formal rules to govern business transactions, there is always a vast margin for leeway, uncertainties, compromises, persuasions and dissimulations. These vary from the brute force of other people's guns and muscles, to one's own personal charm. Magic influence resides in between those two poles, partaking of the qualities of both personal charm and brute force.

In Chapter 1 I related the story of Misha's encounter with a magus from the Centaur centre, when he tried to make her remove the 'little scarf of bad luck' that she saw on his neck. I also mentioned the stone, the tiger eye, she gave him for protection. Even though Misha was turned off by the nonchalant manner in which the amulet was given to him, he kept and cherished the stone for a long time, trying to follow all the instructions he had received from the magus in connection with it. He commented: 'This all acts on the level of the unconscious. If a person is convinced that he is protected, then all the forces of the body are mobilised, just by virtue of this conviction. This stone was all I had in this life to rely on. I had nothing else. The State would not help me. My relatives are far way, and they themselves are up to their ears in trouble. And I have no friends here [in Moscow] – only business partners, and they won't help you. All they'll do is dig you in even deeper – *biznes* is *biznes!*'

In this statement, pronounced matter-of-factly, without bitterness, just stating the situation as it is, Misha implies that what we understand as 'contract', the agreement between parties to a business arrangement, has for him little or no trust-bearing potential. In his words, rather the opposite is true: what he expects from his business partners is that they will try and 'dig him in ever deeper' whenever they get a chance: the game of business is the war of all against all, a walk over a minefield. He recognises that his case is aggravated by his personal situation, because, not having been born in Moscow, he lacks two basic forms of social ties – kinship and friendship – that are by themselves invested by, if not trust per se, then maybe by hope that the individuals involved will not 'dig you in' as a matter of course.

Contract is built on trust in abstract institutions, notions and ideas, but to work in Russia, it must be supplemented by other bonds that command loyalty. Apart from contract, Hart (1988) singled out two other mechanisms that can serve as a basis for economic relations when the 'free' market takes the place of the retreating state with its administrative-command methods. One is that of kinship relations, and the other is that of friendship, a crucial type of human connection everywhere that Hart defined as 'the zone of free-floating social relationships formed by choice, in the expectation of mutuality' (1988: 178). Kinship ties do play a role in Russia as structures of trust: they are ultimate safeguards for survival, connections from which people tend to expect, and sometimes receive, practical help and solidarity that sustain them through difficult moments of life. When millions of state employees were not paid salaries for months, people relied mostly on kinship ties. When a person is severed from the network of kinship ties and thrown into the big city to survive all on his own, he feels totally exposed, as Misha was well aware. But kinship obligations in Soviet times were never really formalised, and in practice they were often weakened; as structures of trust, they were destroyed by the State's ubiquitous surveillance, when brother could inform on brother, and children were encouraged to turn in their parents on ideological grounds. After the end of Stalin's reign of terror, this did not happen often, and the nuclear family grew strong under the subsequent Soviet regime, especially ties between parents and children.

The narrow set of well-defined kinship ties, embracing more often than not only the nuclear family, is too limited to be of importance in providing for the long-standing mutual obligations necessary for market relations. The institution of friendship was the primary base of solidarity in Soviet times (see also Shlapentokh 1989). Kin could well turn up on the other side of the ideological divide in questions of loyalty to the State and attitudes to Soviet ideology, as was often the case in pre-perestroika Russia. Friends, by contrast, one could choose freely. These relationships were seen as free from mercantile considerations (even though, as mentioned above, friendship and *blat* were often inseparable). It was the feeling of choosing freely that gave such value to friendship, exactly as Hart points out for the African migrants he studied (1988). Choosing friends in the Soviet era was one of the few expressions of agency, a free choice, that was left to the Soviet person. Freely chosen friends shared ideological beliefs, artistic preferences, and leisure interests, values and mores, as well as the intricate language codes that marked people from the same social circles.

Friendship ties were heavily charged with obligations, and commitments to friends came before all other social commitments, certainly well before those to the State and its ideology. As I noted above, in Soviet times, friends (and relatives) served as the only source of money-lending, and these credits could be quite substantial, amounting to many years of personal savings. These informal contracts of borrowing were hard to breach due to the high moral value that friendship ties had. In Soviet Russia the individual was never really autonomous in the sense of possessing her own personal time and space, even if she happened to live in an apartment or a room of her own: friends always had right of access to one's space and to one's personal time for as long as they deemed necessary. A friend could call you or pay you a visit, unexpected, at any hour of the day or night, and claim any amount of your time in order to discuss her problems. Friends played the role of psychologists and priests in the confessional. To be without these ties was to be extremely socially vulnerable. This is indicated in Misha's pronouncement concerning the absence of friends: all other, more pragmatically defined, social contacts, will only want to 'dig you in', as he seems to suggest. This is also suggested by the semantics of the terms of affliction discussed in Chapter 2, such as 'the seal of loneliness', the magical diagnosis that implies not only the absence of friends but the inability to acquire them.

With the rise of the market, many a friendship tie was put to the test. In market-driven everyday life, money became its fuel, the new currency that replaced the old one of friendship. The expectations on which friendship had been built, especially their monetary aspects, were often thwarted when one of the parties to the friendship dyad happened to be more successful in generating cash. The changing significance of money altered the fabric of sociality itself. When I returned to Moscow in 1999, the parties of my youth, with lavish food and wine, were largely a thing of the past. People (at least those of my social set) could not afford to buy much food or alcohol, and they were reluctant to receive friends at a meagre table. In the past one had offered what one managed to 'get hold of' (*dostal*). Now it was rather a question of consumer choices – so familiar in the West, but much less so in Russia.

Ledeneva (1998) discusses the changes in the institution of friendship in some detail. According to her data, in 1991–1992 friends were considered the most reliable business partners, while by 1994 the respondents stated that 'friends must be excluded from business, otherwise friendship is lost. If business is run by a friendship, it is not a business' (pp. 195–196). One reason that Ledeneva indicates is that the conditions of the market rule out the instrumental expectations of friendship, spelled out in the rhetoric of mutual help: in Soviet times, the resources distributed among friends were state property, while now they are one's own. Also, the means of solving conflicts in today's business in Russia include harsh measures that most people would be reluctant to apply to their friends. In the words of one of Ledeneva's respondents, the element of trust inherent in friendship gave way to that of rational 'calculation of risks' – 'a specific ethic without morality' (Beck 1992, quoted in Ledeneva 1998: 204). I shall argue below that, whereas trust has indeed disappeared, it is, however, somewhat misleading to speak about Russian business in terms of pure calculation: the social game of business in Russia is indeed a game without rules. In the words of Ledeneva's respondent, a young businessman, 'I was let down, so I let the others down': letting the other down becomes the element of strategy. 'One has to violate one's own principles … The formula of success is to … overcome one's own limits' (ibid.) If the rule of the game is that there are no rules, a statement of the type 'everything can be calculated nowadays, all costs are clear' (ibid.) becomes self-contradictory. The very essence of business life in today's Russia is that there are some things that can not be calculated, and the cost of a mistake can be one's own life.

Among the implicit ontologies that underpin the work of *magi*, there is the notion of the 'money channel', sometimes also referred to as the money code: only those people equipped with this channel (or code) are fit to deal with *biznes* and to make money. There is a range of folk spells and rituals to attract money, not necessarily connected to business activities. But the tacit understanding, as communicated to me unequivocally by Katerina, is that if you are not endowed with the money channel, you should not even consider entering the world of business. There are also channels for excelling in one's professional life; to be successful in a particular occupation, one should possess the corresponding channel. When clients come to a magus with specific complaints concerning their work or business life, a perceptive and conscientious magus will tell a client if he or she has the requisite channel for a profession or business. If the client does have it, and yet her professional life is poor or problem-ridden, the mag can work on that energy-wise (*energeticheski*) and through rituals and spells.

According to this understanding, the ability to make money is a variety of endowment from above, a certain type of magical flow connecting the cosmos and the human being. Indeed, in the life of contemporary Russians, money is the sole prerequisite of any kind of acceptable social existence. It indexes not only relations with the divine power, but also the crucial human connections of kinship, friendship, and even romantic love. (This is my personal observation, but see also Ries 2002.) As noted above, these ties are characterised by material commitments in terms of direct allocations and exchanges of support and services. A person who comes across a decent sum of money is, according to the moral system of pre-perestroika times, expected, or maybe even morally compelled, to infuse his or her close ties with 'monetary energy'. This is undoubtedly so in the ties of romantic love, where the force of feeling is (often) directly indexed by, and evaluated through, the amount of money and commodities that are invested in the tie (canonically in man's love to woman, but the opposite can also be true, as we saw in the case of Liuba and her husband). It is this indexing that makes it possible for the agents to compare the emotional intensities of these various ties, in the colloquial terms of 'whom he loves more', and that adds fuel to fires of jealousy and hatred that often accompany the various affective bonds. (Recall Tolia's mother in Chapter 3 who complained that her older son showered his wife with money and presents, while the more basic kinship tie, that with his mother, was undernourished). Conflicts over money and property are among the most common situations where magic is used.

Lack of money, and the pressing need to earn it, is a constant strain in Russian everyday life. The gaps between the haves and have-nots are evident in food, clothing, living conditions, quality of health care, child care and education, leisure time, and more (see also Humphrey 2002b, Ch. 9). People living on a pension or on the salary of a school or a kindergarten teacher, a factory worker, or an employee of one of the multitude of bureaucratic establishments, including law-enforcement bodies, feel humiliated and deprived, especially when they remember how opportunities were equal only a couple decades ago. Marrying, bringing up a child, giving a passed-away parent a decent burial, arranging a simple birthday party, or having coffee with a friend in one of Moscow's numerous and well-supplied cafés becomes problematic for a person living only on state wages.

This social exclusion feels all the more bitter since the have-nots are constantly exposed to the world of the haves. One of the symbols of the world of the rich is a flashy Mercedes speeding through the streets in violation of all traffic rules. A joke has it that if one drives a Mercedes one does not even need to look at the road; indeed, I can confirm that this joke has a strong basis in reality. Having money means being beyond the law, people say; while this same 'law', embodied by policemen, resentfully called '*menty*', or the traffic police, *gaishniki* (the officers of *GAI*, the State Automobile Inspectorate) are constantly expected to harass the rest, extorting money from the public to supplement their own meagre living. The profusion of goods and services that are desirable, efficient and of good quality is painfully visible and readily available to both relations and friends who are better off. As such, they only accentuate the humiliation experienced by those who, for one reason or another, did not make it.

It was not clear to Misha why he was so afflicted by loneliness, betrayal, and bad luck. He was an amiable, good-looking young man, he was prepared to work hard, he did not expect favours from the world, and he was open to creating bonds of friendship. But all his ties turned out to be *biznes* companions rather than friends. The way they treated him, they only confirmed his view of business companionship as a variety of grave-digging. They certainly ruled out any possibility of trust, and they hardly left any space for hope.

There are a number of colloquial expressions in today's Russian language to connote various types of violence, extortion and monetary fraud that people can fall prey to in their public and professional life. These expressions are new in popular speech, probably borrowed from the criminal underground, with its own rich folklore and mythology, and not entirely devoid of romantic aura for the peaceful citizens outside its borders. One popular word, '*naezd*' (verb: *naezzhat'*) has already been discussed above. *Naezd* (raid) can be connected with claims of large sums of money that the 'driving' side threatens to extort from the victim under threat of violence.

There are more slang words for the ways in which a person can be made to part with his money. One can be 'thrown on money' (*kinut' na den'gi*). In this case, one suffers a one-time loss as a result of one's credulity – for example, when one does not get paid for work performed, or when a wholesaler puts money upfront for a consignment of goods and gets neither goods nor money back (or, conversely, when one delivers goods but never gets paid, as happened to Nina's husband Valerii in Chapter 5).

Misha was 'thrown on money' repeatedly, as, for example, when he himself received the money for the consignment (in that particular case it was German canned beer). He then gave this money to his companion for safe-keeping, awaiting the day when the suppliers would come to claim their share. The companion, however, disappeared with all the money, and all trace of him vanished somewhere around Germany (maybe the correspondence with the origin of the goods was not coincidental, pointing to the fact that the whole operation had been premeditated). Misha was left to be hunted for many months by the armed men that the furious suppliers sent after him.

Another possible pitfall in this category Misha managed to avoid, since it requires that the victim should have a decent fortune to begin with. The trick is called '*razvesti na den'gi*'. *Razvesti* means to make one part with someone or something, to divorce, dissolve or dilute, but *razvodit'* also means to breed, rear or cultivate. This is when a person is swindled into investing a large sum of money in an enterprise, and is left with nothing. In this case, the victim is 'divorced' or parted from his money, but he can also be seen figuratively as an agricultural species especially bred by the 'croppers' so as to yield a one-time harvest. Still worse, one can be 'hooked on money' (*posadit' na den'gi*) as one is 'hooked on the needle' (*posadit' na iglu*) when one becomes addicted to a narcotic drug. In this case a person is drawn into a business project and is forced, by coercion or cunning, to pay again and again, until he is stripped of all his assets. A more severe variety of this is to be 'set on the counter' (*postavit' na schetchik*), when someone is faced with the choice between paying the sum immediately or accepting the final count-down on his life. Serezha's father, in the case described in Chapter 3, was 'set on the counter', as his widow told me, but he managed to project the kinship curse onto his son, before his time was up.

When I met Misha, he had just been 'thrown on money' most unceremoniously. He had recently completed the renovation of several flights of stairs in a five-storey apartment block. He had had a verbal agreement (a sort of a contract) with a municipal official. Misha had been apprehensive about doing such a big job without any written guarantees, but he was dissuaded from this by the official status of his contractor, not only a holder of an official post, but also an elected municipal politician (a *deputat* of the local council). When Misha finished the job and went to his employer to get paid, the official was no longer there, and his successor was unwilling to pay for assignments issued by someone else. Misha was told that he might be paid from the next quarter's budget, but he received no guarantees. This was a typical case where people with a stronger degree of protection ('*krysha*') would resort to the help of the 'muscle men in leather jackets with shaven heads', as Misha put it. But at the time he had no such protection.

This put-down happened when he had been carrying Zinaida's stone for quite some time, around the time when he felt that all his troubles were getting worse by the day, thickening like a cloud. By then, he had already been giving me lifts for several months, and this was the moment when I introduced him to Katerina, the event that for him proved to be the turning-point of his life.

After looking at Misha and consulting her cards, Katerina asked him if there was an older woman in his life who wished him ill. Misha, thinking of his wife, readily confirmed that there was such a woman. Katerina told him that his wife had tried to do a *privorot* on him after he had left and she had realised that he was not coming back. Being present at this first diagnostic séance, I silently questioned this, remembering that the wife herself had practically thrown Misha out, inflicting on him such an *obida* that he had no choice but to leave. But who could fathom a woman's heart? Misha did not seem to find any incongruity in Katerina's diagnosis; in fact, he seemed to endorse it completely, and, in general, he was perceptibly taken in by Katerina's charisma. She told him that his wife had used magic to bring him back, but this was weak, amateurish work, which had not achieved the desired end, but managed to do considerable harm to Misha's bio-field. 'Do you have any photographs of her?' she asked. No, Misha admitted that his wife had been very careful not to leave any photos of her in his possession.

'She knew what she was doing', concluded Katerina, 'She was indeed someone who knew about magic.'

After Katerina's first treatment, Misha was a changed man. Before the séance, Katerina had asked him 'to relax and not to think about anything'. He tried the best he could. 'She must be able to read my thoughts', he said to me afterwards. 'Every time I started to think about something, she sighed deeply: she knew! And she told me that my wife's *privorot* had not only blocked my upper channel, but it also perforated my bio-field: it was the beginning of *porcha*, she saw this when she was working with my [energo-information] structures. She pointed out where exactly this perforation (*proboi*) was – on the left side of my shoulder blade. And every time she concentrated on that place, I felt a stabbing sensation (*prokol*), as if I had been shot through by an electric current or by a big needle.'

Despite the pain, after this séance Misha was totally euphoric. His eyes glittered, and his mood was akin to deep elation. 'I don't remember when I last felt so happy', he said to me, 'Now I know for sure that everything will be fine. The main thing is to know that there is someone covering your back, someone who is on your side.' I wondered why he did not ask her to help him get paid for the staircase renovation work left after the disappearance of the deputy to the municipal council. He said that he did not want to bother her with such trifles: he felt that she was bearing all the burdens of the world on her fragile shoulders, and he did not want to add to it with his trivial problems. 'There will be more jobs', he said with conviction, 'Money is rubbish, I feel that money will come my way now.'

Misha started visiting Katerina regularly, twice a week. He was still living with his Indian friends, earning the bare essentials of life by driving his old car. But now he received some new orders for renovation jobs. Some of them were mediated by Katerina; others turned up as if from nowhere. Other offers, more in the nature of business deals, also came his way. This was when Misha really needed Katerina's help. The ruthless interpersonal combat of wills that is sometimes involved in a complex business deal requires careful monitoring. Walking a tightrope (or a mine field) is made easier if there is someone standing on the side with a safety pole. Even with a safety arrangement, every step can be your last, but this safety arrangement is what makes every next step possible, preventing the paralysing effect of fear on a person's psyche and body.

Elsewhere (Lindquist 2000b) I have discussed the work of magic in business, based on the example of another of Katerina's clients: a middle-aged woman who tried to make her way in the world of Moscow's petty commerce. For other types of business, the conditions are much the same, although combinations can vary in scale and in degree of complexity. Generally, people who make it big must have an initial access to the structures of distribution and decision making. However, in addition, they must be innovative in their thinking and have luck on their side. There follow some of the schemes or 'combinations' (*kombinatsii*) that I heard about from various people in Moscow.[2]

1. The State has to pay salaries to miners in a city in the Urals. The State does not have the money, but it does have income from customs dues. A state employee is instructed to collect money from customs dues that come from a large consignment of imported goods, and remit it to the miners. The Urals are far away from Moscow, and the miners' factory has no connections with the customs office, and so it is far from easy to check how much money from this operation ends up in the pocket of the civil servant.

2. Humanitarian aid is a lucrative source of income for people who are integrated in the corresponding structures. Humanitarian help comes in several forms. One is goods and equipment, for example, medicines, disposable syringes or quick chemical test-sets, clothes, toys, or household appliances for orphanages, retirement-homes and hospitals. Another form is goods and foodstuffs intended for sale in the regular retail network, in state- or municipal-owned stores (which still exist side by side with privately owned ones). These goods are not liable to customs duties paid by the buyers, and the income from their sale is not taxed. Goods labelled as 'humanitarian aid' proceed from the customs to warehouses, where they are placed under the responsibility of the specialised charity funds. To organise such a fund, connections at a high level of political decision making are required, and the directors of these funds are free to handle the goods. These transactions are subjected to control, however: every once in a while, an inspection commission can come and demand papers confirming that the humanitarian aid has reached the

targeted consignees, be it a boarding school for deaf children, a foster-home, or a hospital in a provincial town. Fund directors sell part of the merchandise and receive payment for it. They must 'arrange' the necessary papers with the target receiving establishment, the papers that will show that the goods have reached their intended destination. The director of the orphanage etc., produces such papers (not free of charge, of course). The merchandise is then sold to those who pay. The fund director must have connections with the wholesale buyers and it is he who gets the money from selling the goods. For the wholesale buyers, papers must be arranged attesting to the fact that the goods have come from suppliers (in most cases foreign), and that they have been properly cleared by customs.

3. A good source of big and quick money is licensing. A person with connections in the licensing department has an idea that wine under a certain brand name will sell well. Let's say that this brand name corresponds to a popular football club, or to a well-known geographical locality. The person contacts the people who are entitled to sell the football-club brand name, and persuades them to sell it to her. She contacts the producers, who pay for the brand name. She quotes different amounts of money to the buyer and the seller; the difference is what she puts in her own pocket. Or, she buys wine from a foreign producer for a certain amount of money, but quotes a much higher amount to the buyer to whom she sells the wine in Moscow. The difference, again, is hers. Good money may be made on customs dues, when the business person quotes one sum for the dues to the buyer but agrees on a much lower one with a customs officer in charge of the particular batch of goods. The customs officer gets his share of the difference, and the rest goes to the businessperson as pure revenue. In Russian colloquial speech this revenue is called '*navar*', the top layer of a pot of soup that has been boiling for some time and which contains all the goodness.

4. Representatives of the new bodies of power, especially members of parliament, have many ways of getting rich during the relatively short period when they are entrusted with the honour of being the people's representatives. (These are the members of the Duma, about whom many a joke has been circulating since this democratic institution started its work of legislation and rule.)

One of them is standing as guarantor for the purchase or sale of property. Another is selling apartments that Duma members obtained in service. A major source of income is financial operations through banks. Let us say there is a large construction order whose contractor is the municipality of Moscow (as in the case with Godfather in Misha's story). The Moscow municipal budget allocates several million dollars for building an office complex, a sports facility, a monastery, or a school. The person in charge of the project sells it to the highest bidder. A construction company applies to a bank for a loan. It undertakes to repay by instalments, the first payment due in a year's time. It is up to the manager of the bank to make the decision whether to grant the loan or not. The manager will feel safer in future if such a loan request is supported by a letter of guarantee from a Duma member or from the Moscow municipality (for this letter, the contractor is prepared to pay very good money; a large sum goes to pay the bank manager for the favourable decision). The money of the clients of the bank goes to the contractor (people like Godfather), and a percentage might go to the author of the 'combination', if he or she is not the same person as the contractor himself. The bank gives all its money to the contractor, and in a year's time it claims bankruptcy. There is nothing the law can do to punish the bank manager, who by that time might be far way in Cyprus or the Maldives with his money. The clients of the bank can do nothing, except for hiring muscle-men in leather jackets, to find the bank manager and to 'put him on the counter'. But the muscle-men's services are expensive and can be afforded only by a few.

5. The Moscow Energy Department provides energy to the subway system, for which the subway managers are supposed to pay the Energy Department. The subway system is funded by the State. The State owes money to workers drilling oil in the north-west of Russia. Someone within the Energy Department arranges it so that the energy goes directly to the subway system, and the subway manager remits money directly to the oil drillers. The difference goes to the person within the Energy Department who has made the arrangement, who may or may not be the author of the scheme. In the latter case, a share of the 'navar' goes to the author.

More examples could be adduced. Some of them beggar belief, others are too complicated to follow. But schemes like this must be operating, since there is no other way of accounting for the large numbers of very rich people when compared with the poverty of those who live on their salaries, or on their income from 'private entrepreneurship'. Such 'projects' need a clear and well-structured mind, and intimate acquaintance with how various mechanisms work. They require systemic thinking, good protection in case something goes wrong (meaning people in high positions in the judiciary and the law-enforcement system and possibly also in the criminal world), flexible performance, and a high degree of social competence. Numbers of people must be brought together, many subtle combinations must be worked through. The organiser of such a scheme must possess a great deal of persuasiveness and self-assurance. He or she must have flawless social skills in dealing with various people on various levels: customs officers, bankers, miners' representatives, state inspectors, retailers, directors of orphanages, and many others. All these people must be interested in the project, reassured against possible setbacks, and motivated to cooperate. Some of them must be befriended to be persuaded to do what they are asked, or to feel safe to take a bribe or to take part in the scheme for the future share of the revenue. They must be ensured against fall-outs from aggressive attacks, against *naezdy*, if a person at some node of the web suddenly demands more money than was agreed on. Every failure can entail heavy casualties for many persons involved: patrons, friends, husbands and lovers, the latter two categories often intimately entangled in the machinery of these business transactions for the female actors. The 'combinators' must be protected from above in case something goes wrong, and they must be able to disappear without trace when it is over. A quick and cold mind, audacity and apt decision making are all imperative not only for the progress of business, but often also for the physical survival of the author of the combination, and maybe of her immediate entourage.

The magus is used as a consultant to make the requisite decisions. Clients may discuss the project with the magus at the stage of conception, when they ask her to 'examine' it (*prosmotret'*, literally, to look it over, to see its potentialities and pitfalls). The magus is usually not initiated into the details of the operation, the names of the organisations, the actual persons involved, or the type of the merchandise in the deal. The initial request may be extremely vague. The magus is informed that there is a prospect of a business operation, and asked to check if it is worthwhile to embark on. She starts by looking into her cards, offering tentative details that are confirmed or rejected by the client. For example:

'I see a man there, on quite a high level, not on the very highest, but close to it. He is also involved with the force structures.[3] His protection is crucial for the outcome of the whole plan. He must be given some additional private interest in the case in order to ensure his involvement. If you fail to engage this man, it is better not to start the whole thing at all.' – 'Yes, this is my former lover and good friend, he worked in KGB before, but now he is high up in FSB structures' (FSB is the abbreviation for Federal Security Service, an organisation that replaced KGB).

Katerina told me with great reluctance that she does sometimes work with big business. Here is where she, as well as all other magi I worked with, became very reticent: these are 'serious' people who want to remain anonymous, and who are not to be played with. I heard that big business units are entities with their own coherent 'energy structure', and it is these energy structures that the magus or the urban shaman works with (neo-shamaness described in Lindquist 2002b calls these entities the 'souls of business'). In small and medium-size businesses, however, one deals with specific individuals, with their agendas, needs and desires, and it is on this level that the work of magic operates.

Misha's life improved considerably after he met Katerina. He was able to leave his Indian friends and move, once again, into a rented apartment. Later, he realised his old dream and became a real-estate agent (in the modern Russian, *rieltor*). This profession is in high demand in Moscow, bearing in mind the centrality of 'living space' (*zhilploshchad'*) in people's lives. The profession of real-estate agent had existed in Soviet times: the modest and half-shady figure of the 'apartment broker', *kvartirnyi makler*. This was the person who helped people come up with options and schemes to solve the thorny problems of moving apart as well as moving in together. After perestroika, the privatisation of apartments became a source of total confusion: of enrichment for some, total ruination and destruction for others (when alcoholics or old people sold their rights to apartments, for example, and then suddenly found themselves in the street, homeless, or, worse, their relatives simply found them dead). Real-estate dealers became one of the new professions that could provide a decent living without being a criminal, part of the seedbed of a budding new middle class.

Misha found a companion who invited him to cooperate in a scheme. They located a communal apartment, shared by several families, often down-and-out drunkards and impoverished pensioners, and offered them individual apartments in the new residential areas of Moscow (the dream of many who live in communal flats). These apartments were purchased in advance with the money provided by investors and procured by the companion, a man with connections. A large, old apartment in the centre of Moscow, emptied of its tenants, was then sold for the market price, and the revenue was divided between the investors and the companions, of which Misha was one.

This was the job Misha really liked: dealing with people whom he had to convince, dispel their apprehensions, switching on his natural charm, interacting with people on a personal level; driving around Moscow fixing things and striking deals, meeting a host of challenges, both major and minor. It reminded him of the good old days when he was responsible for supply in the Bread Ministry and flew around the whole country achieving small feats of 'getting things done'. People would often have fits of mini-breakdowns when they realised that they were leaving their dwellings for good. 'One of them seized hold of the tap to the mains water-supply in the flat (*vodoprovodnyi kran*), and wrenched it off, simply because he could not come to terms with the idea of leaving; the water flooded the place and eventually warped the wooden flooring, thus ruining the flat altogether ... Another disappeared on the day I waited for him to sign the papers ... As an estate-agent (*rieltor*), one has to be a psychologist, a strategist, a judge of human character, even a bit of a *mag*!' One such operation was done with amazing success, and with the close involvement of Katerina at every step; the partner, however, laid claim to a much bigger sum than had been agreed upon in the beginning, a quarrel ensued, and Misha had to leave the business he liked so much and return to erratic building jobs.

All the while he was totally dependent on his old car in which he would cover the long distances required by his building contracts as well as his real-estate endeavours. When all else failed, he would also use this car to earn money as an unofficial taxi driver. I have described Misha's car in Chapter 1 – its radiator was decorated with the portrait of the Incomparable Cosmic Master Raisa Ryk, to give Misha hope that the car would start next time he put the key in the ignition. This was a hope with precious little foundation in reality, given the parlous state of the splendid old vehicle. But this small miracle somehow happened every day, even if the car was broken into on the parking lot, even if its wheels fell off during the rides, and the window-screen wipers refused to work. Misha's most urgent life-project was to buy another car, a decent used one, for which he was setting aside 1000 dollars. If he were really lucky, he could sell the old car for a couple of hundred dollars, an operation for which people routinely resort to the help of their magi. Misha got a spell from Katerina for this purpose, one he would resort to along with others every morning when he started the car. He even found a buyer who was interested but still undecided.

As in Europe, car owners in Russia have to put their vehicles through regular technical inspections to obtain a certificate testifying to the fact that they are road-worthy. This precious document must be kept close at hand by every driver. At any moment, one can be stopped by the traffic police, because the car is dirty, because the driver does not have his seat-belt on, or for no reason at all. In this case the driver is required to show this certificate, together with the driver's licence and the paper certifying that the driver is the owner of the car (or, failing this, a *doverennost'*, a statement to the effect that the car is entrusted by the owner to the driver). If a driver lacks a valid certificate, if it is overdue or not in order, the driver faces the choice of either paying the police on the spot or forfeiting his driver's licence. Either way, once the driver is stopped by the traffic police, the *GAIshnik*, he must count on having to pay, because there will always be some rules or regulations he has violated. If there are none, the police can always say that the driver was exceeding the speed limit, and the latter has no way of disproving it. Driving in Moscow is always a gamble. By and large, the cars that are stopped are usually those of people like Misha, struggling to survive to the next day with the help of this same car. The Mercedes of New Russians usually do not bother to stop, I am told, and the officers of the *GAI* make no attempt to stop them, knowing full well that they will be up against a higher power. For this reason, the

GAI extortions may well entail an evening without food for most drivers and their families. There are several spells that people put on their cars in order to make them invisible to the *GAI*, to divert the officer's attention somewhere else (maybe to other passing cars).

There are many cars on the streets of Moscow that, like Misha's, would not stand a chance of passing a technical inspection. Like everything else, these certificates can be bought for reasonable money from the people who carry out the inspection, through appropriate mediators, and this is what Misha had done. But one day he was stopped by a traffic policeman, who took one look at his certificate and told Misha that it was forged. 'Look, you are in trouble', the police said, 'False certificates are like false money, a criminal offence liable to years in prison.' 'What shall I do,' pleaded Misha, 'All I have on me is twenty dollars.' 'Are you implying I take bribes?' the policeman asked, 'Leave your papers here and just get lost, you bastard! Soon, you'll be sent for!' Misha drove away, devastated, and called Katerina in panic. She answered calmly that she did not see any real problem about the incident. 'Get hold of fifty dollars and return to the place immediately'.

And indeed, when he soon returned to the policeman and meekly offered him fifty dollars, the policeman was very friendly. He silently took the money and hid it in his pocket, telling Misha that it was very dangerous to drive with a false certificate. The two had a pleasant chat, and the policeman even offered his help in getting a real, genuine certificate, for only 150 dollars, but Misha declined. He was about to sell the car anyway, and such an investment seemed unnecessary. After that, he was careful to use Katerina's spells every time he drove, and it worked well for two more months, while the buyer evaporated into thin air. Then the car suddenly exploded while he was driving, exuding smoke in the midst of the traffic, and he counted himself lucky to be able to park it at the curb and climb out of it, hastily, before it expired in front of his eyes, giving off a plume of black smoke. He had the feeling that he had lost a true friend, but Katerina reassured him that it was a good sign. At the moment, he was getting involved in a real-estate business on a new level. A big company accepted him on probation and sent him to courses in finance and law, and he was full of hope and expectations for the future. He said it was just as well he used public transport, so that nothing would divert him from his studies.

In Katerina's understanding and that of other practitioners, the concerted efforts of the magus and client, reinforced by props and instruments such as spells and rituals, work to change the 'energo-information structures' that are responsible for the more tangible 'structures': both those of the body and those of the social environment of the client and her close ones. What these structures are and how they change remains an open question. What is definitely changed, however, are the structures of subjectivity of at least some clients. For some of them these changes are felt as exceptionally deep and dramatic. In Misha's story, the sense of the new beginning he experienced after meeting Katerina was formulated with remarkable clarity. He felt protected, taken care of, he felt there was someone he could finally rely on; he felt that there was one person who was not there to 'dig you in', but who was prepared to share with you the effort of tramping through the mine-field of Russian life. Misha conveyed this subjectivity of an inordinate effort when he would speak about the burden of responsibility that used to lie on his shoulders 'like a heap of stones', draining him and preventing him from moving further. In his narration, he had another specific way of conveying this change of subjectivity that the work of magic effected in him: through his relationship to the Church.

Like many Russian people who were born in Soviet times, Misha had no meaningful contact with the Church before perestroika. Recall that he was christened at the behest of his austere grandmother, but, apart from the presence of 'screaming small children' he had no real recollection of the event. Later in life, having married and moved to Moscow, he had another encounter with the Church. This was when he was commissioned by his wife to be a guide for a couple of visitors from remote provinces. 'They wanted to see a church, to be present at the liturgy, and I had to take them there, although I did not feel like it at all. As we approached the church, I was overcome by reluctance, as if my legs refused to carry me. When I entered and tried to make the sign of the cross, I felt dizzy and sick, and almost fell, and I had to go out and wait in the car while they continued with their sightseeing.' This was his first and last visit to church in many years, until he started to go to Katerina and follow the detailed instructions for his treatment with which she endeavoured to improve his life.

Apart from 'energy work', spells and rituals, a central part of the treatment that Katerina demands of all who become her permanent clients is to start to engage more closely with the Church. They are required to stand through the liturgy and go to Eucharist, as an absolute minimum. This is considered the primary purifying and energising measure, without which Katerina's continued energy work is deemed less than effective. (I must note here that this element of treatment is included only for ethnic Russians with a working-class background. Katerina never required this from, for example, ethnic Jews or Tatars, nor of Western Europeans when she had to work with them, nor from the representatives of the academic intelligentsia, who, according to her keen social intuition, would have a hostile and contemptuous attitude to the Church.)

Misha started to go to church services, and stood through them overwhelmed with illumination. He left church with a light heart, as if his unshiftable burden (*nosha nepod'emnaia*) had been miraculously removed. 'The smells, the sounds, the colours, it was so full of beauty, and I was a part of it ... This beauty filled my heart, lifting my load, lifting myself over the ground. I think these were amongst the happiest moments in my life. I had a feeling that the door was open. I felt that tomorrow was there for me to enter, as it would be into Heaven' (*Zavtra bylo otkryto dla menia, ia mog v nego voiti kak v tsarstvie nebesnoie'*).

In a society where 'societal hope' (Hage 2003) is scarce, there must exist other ways to secure a temporal dimension for an individual struggling to play this society's cruel social games. Where structural dimensions of agency are limited, alternative practices offer its affective dimension, the possibility of hope. The subjectivity of hope, vividly expressed by Misha as 'the door opened into tomorrow', is naturally expressed in the religious feelings that overwhelm the person in precisely those areas which formerly had seemed the darkest and most oppressive. These religious revelations, experienced in the context of an encounter with the magus, are for the clients linked with the aura of the magus's personality, indexically transmitting divine power through the figure of the magus on to that of the client, endowing the client with the channels of agency and with a subjective feeling of strength. In the language of the native cultural ontologies, 'the channels open up and the energy flows'. These are some of the ways of conveying the emotional state of an individual who was given back the chance to keep his *illusio*: who has been given hope.

In 2004 I come to Moscow from time to time. Misha meets me in the airport, for old times' sake. I never pay him for these rides any more. It would be awkward, even insulting, to offer payment for going in this latest-model, brand-new Toyota. Admittedly, it is neither a Mercedes nor a Jeep, brands connoting even greater money and status; but Misha is quite content with his new car. For this one he does not need any spells: it starts instantly, it is never robbed at its paid parking place, and it is never stopped by the traffic police, regardless of how fast he drives. He gave me his new business card: he's now the head of a real-estate company, in charge of a couple of dozen people. He is not Misha anymore: people call him Mikhail Mikhailovich. But it is fine for me to call him Misha; and he now calls me by my first name and by the second person singular, 'na ty'. Misha is a respected businessman these days, and he can afford to treat me as an equal. On our long rides from the airport, sitting in the interminable traffic jams, I still enjoy our chats, as he tells me stories about business life in the great metropolis. Yet his stories have become vague and empty of content: the more 'serious' your business, the less you should talk. I tried to probe the nature of his activities nowadays – I tell him I don't care for particulars, what I'd like to hear are general patterns of how things are done – but he lets nothing slip. I recognise this reticence from other people who deal with more substantial business: at some point I'll face a blank wall, even with the best of informants. Instead, Misha recounts fondly, though with some irony, his business breakfasts in luxury hotels with the Lions club, whose member he has become. He likes the atmosphere of the business breakfasts, even though he doesn't think much of the club's charitable projects. Otherwise, conversations with Misha now are less ethnographic excursions, more samples of the rhetoric of a 'self-made man', which he undoubtedly is. Misha and Katerina have parted company, and, in his didactic monologues on the worth of having done it all by himself, there is not a word acknowledging Katerina's contribution.

I know that this is always the case, but still it makes me sad. I am grateful to Misha for meeting me in the airport – taxi drivers in Sheremetievo are real sharks – and I admire his achievements. Still, I remember the old Misha of my fieldwork with some nostalgia – his old car, his spells against the traffic police, his elation after Katerina's séances, his ardent admiration for his magus. He is on the crest of the wave now, even though he admits that business life in Moscow is as perilous a minefield as it ever was. Will he turn to other magi at some later point? My sense is that, if he does, he won't tell me anymore.

Notes.

1. This occupation, unofficially known as '*tolkach*', was described in Ledeneva (1998). A curious transmutation of *blat*, it was based on the use of private connections for the good of the enterprise, instead of using the official or job connections for one's private sake, as is otherwise the case in *blat*).

2. Detailed information on protection racket and security companies is found in Volkov (2000) and in other contributions to Ledeneva and Kurkchiyan (2000); and in Humphrey (2002b, Ch. 5).

3. Force structures' (*silovye struktury*) are a conglomerate of law-enforcement structures that can, by definition, solve problems through the use of force. They include state and private police and security forces, the latter being a recent transformation of the informal 'protection' groups also known as 'racketeers' or 'mafia'.

Epilogue
Social Fields, Fields of the Game, Minefields: Hazards of Interpretation

I embarked on this work with a vague sense of dissatisfaction with the epistemological strategy of cultural interpretation which is basic to much anthropological writing. The guiding trope of enquiry was, for me, not the Geertzian project of 'interpretation of cultures' but, rather, Bourdieu's notion of the 'logic of practice'. In order to discern this logic, I attempted to account for 'meeting face-to-face' with the Other, not translating the Other in the terms of the self, but showing why some ways of thinking and being were logical within the frames of certain practices, social contexts, or 'fields of the game'. I started to unravel this logic from one specific cultural domain, that of magic and healing. The concept of 'the logic of practice' is connected with other useful notions that Bourdieu offered later: 'social field', which he also referred to as 'field of the game', and *illusio*, the stakes made in this game. All these terms can be seen as so many attempts to find a standpoint for the student of the life of the Other to secure a view from inside instead of from outside; not to interpret the Other in the language of the Self, but to imagine what it would be like for the Self to play the same game as the Other, which means, among other things, to engage in the same processes of interpretation.

In my field, I tried to approach this logic of practice in terms of patterns of signification: to decode this logic as cultural semiosis, understood as signs acting on people, and as people producing and interpreting signs. In the end, interpretation thus emerged as central to this book, even though what I tried to do was not to interpret the world of the Other into a different set of terms, but, instead, to follow people's own interpretations. Along the way, I ended up doing more interpretation than I ever imagined I would need. Several Russian words, crucial for the understanding of the logic of practice, simply could not be rendered through any direct interpretation, but needed long explication with excursions into this very practice. The worlds of meanings are untranslatable in an exact one-to-one mode; we are only imaginable for each other insofar as we meet face to face, which implies engaging in the same dynamics of signification, plugging into the same semiotic chains. These chains have their consistent, although possibly sometimes fuzzy logic, and to be able to follow this logic was for me the enjoyment of the meeting with the Other. This enjoyment, I realised, comes from seeing the ways in which human agency always manages to find channels through which to manifest itself; the ways in which human sociality always operates, bypassing the most intractable structures of enslavement and impossibility. The enjoyment was to see how, out of the misery of historical turmoil and transformations, in situations of deep uncertainty and lack of control, agency and imagination conjure up ways for hope to materialise: to congeal desire, to balance off uncertainty by providing a time dimension, to create a tomorrow, a future to strive for.

I attempted to capture this forward thrust by using the notion of hope. For the people I talked to, hope was an existential doorway out of the deadliest of deadlocks, the light at the end of the longest of tunnels; a tool for expanding the horizons of the life-world, for intentionality to unfold, for will to return: the will to life, no matter what. In worlds where selves are constructed with no hard and fast boundaries separating them from one another, and where consciousness is conceived as continuous with the body, 'human beings are wizards to each other, and social life is at first magical' (Sartre 1948: 84, quoted in Kapferer 1997). Consciousness is both embodied and constituted through signs. It is therefore no wonder that men and women can make and unmake each other using as weapons signs that are culturally conceived as potent, be it material objects, words, gestures or other movements, units of ritual, poetry, or other kinds of semiotic complexes.

Words, as well as the other signs we use, are not innocent: they are heavily loaded with presuppositions, intellectual as well as sensual and emotional. They guide us along the trails of semiosis in certain directions, and they are anchored in certain ontologies of which we are often unaware. I suppose my use of semiosis, with its ensuing emphasis on interpretation, could make me vulnerable to accusations of excessive intellectualism: decoding signs is associated with rationalist activities, while most of this book deals with emotions, passions, desires, and the ailments of the body. Also, the very term 'practice' presupposes activities performed unthinkingly, somewhat removed from purposeful calculation and deliberate consideration. As Bourdieu has put it, practice is in-the-body, as well as in the dispositions that are beyond rationality and calculating awareness. Practice, of which interpretation is an intrinsic and continuous part, involves the processes of semiosis. In semiosis as envisaged by Peirce, and illustrated by magical practices described in this book, signs, and especially their Objects and Interpretants, can lie outside the sphere of the rational and intellectual. Signs, and 'trafficking' with them, include as much bodily perceptions as they do emotions, desires and passions – the stuff of the psyche (or heart, or soul, whatever the culture in question would choose to call the realm of their provenance).

In this concluding section, I shall undertake a reverse type of exercise from what I have been attempting in the previous pages. Instead of unweaving the shared semiotic ground for key 'indigenous' terms, I shall try to test two notions that Western social science often uses unproblematically as neutral, universally applicable, analytical terms: those of risk and trust.

Two institutions that are basic to Western society are market and democracy. These are the very institutions that are considered to be the pillars of Western life, making it 'free', in contrast to 'dictatorships', 'autocracies', and 'totalitarian regimes'. Reforms attempting to introduce these two basic institutions into the post-Soviet reality were the initial conditions on which the West was prepared to start recognising post-Communist Russia both as an equal partner on the international arena – a partner for cooperation instead of confrontation – and as a recipient for all possible sorts of aid, subsidies and donations from Western donors.

Contract and competition, and thus trust and risk, are intrinsic to the functioning of both these institutions. Risk involves challenge and unpredictability, and is based on the realisation that advantages, be it profit or excitement, are to be gained only if something is at stake. Trust in abstract institutions is a *sine qua non* for any conceivable system of democracy at large. In addition, trust in a business partner, as well as in the systems of laws and regulations hedging off the unpredictability that the market is fraught with – balancing off risk – is indispensable for the operation of market mechanisms in any form. Risk and trust are implied even in Bourdieu's seemingly neutral notion 'the field of the game' (under which institutions of both market and democracy can be subsumed). The game has something at stake – what Bourdieu calls *illusio* – and thus presupposes risk; and, to be able to play at all, the players must have trust that the basic rules of the game will not change without notification, and that the other players will abide by these rules.

In the West, risk is controlled partly by legal mechanisms; partly it is balanced by trust in abstract institutions as well as in concrete individuals. Trust makes both contract and competition possible. But what of the life of Misha, Katerina, Anna, Nina, and other people encountered in this book? What of a society where the social institutions that should be trusted are instead feared, despised and ridiculed? We have seen that the representatives of the official structures of the State are considered 'real beasts'; they can be dealt with only on a one-to-one, face-to-face basis, when they become concrete individuals instead of representatives of abstract institutions, and can thus become enmeshed in the networks of personalised exchange of gifts, favours, and possibly even human warmth and mutual assistance.

This assistance, however, is based on something other than contract, and involves, as I shall try to show in a moment, something other than what is meant in the West by 'trust'. And what are the consequences if such ties fail? The stories of the people presented here indicate that 'risk' is not a suitable concept either: what is at stake is not loss at a game; instead, it is different degrees of collapse of the whole life-edifice, demolition of the life-world *in toto*. What in the Western world would be thought of as a breach of contract, is here conceptualised by a strong word, 'betrayal' (*predatel'stvo*). What in the West would be dealt with through legal means of punishment and through the networks of insurance and state welfare, is here managed by the help of muscle men (if one is lucky enough to have access to them) or, more affordably, with the help of magic.

Luhmann (1988) remarks that individuals concern themselves with probabilities, and the highly probable has a tendency to be normalised. As we have seen, in the personal and professional lives of people in Russia the probability of being let down is exceedingly high, while the consequences are dire and sometimes even lethal (being killed by hired guns for having no money to pay back a loan; dying in a hospital with no one to take care of you; losing your son in the military if you have no contacts and no money to pay bribes). Whereas suffering and death may never be experienced as 'normal', in a situation where they are recurrent they inevitably become part of what Luhmann calls the 'familiar'. For a person like Misha, Anna or Olga, or a small trader I described elsewhere (see Lindquist 2000b), their disaster threshold must be higher than for their comparable Western counterparts. (I recall here the sneers of my Russian guests visiting Sweden and hearing Swedes complain about 'stress' and other hardships of life. Being a part of what Nancy Ries would call a genre of talk (1997), this contemptuous attitude to the everyday suffering of Westerners has something to do with the realities, normalities and disaster thresholds that can not be compared.)

Let me, for the last time in this book, attempt an exercise in interpretation, and compare the semantic fields of the terms 'trust' and 'risk' with those of their Russian counterparts. Risk is directly translated into the Russian word *risk*, and the meaning of this word is largely the same as in English. What is different, however, is the cultural attitude to risk in Russia which is, by and large, much more enthusiastic than that in the West. In the West, people realise that risk is increasingly present in society, but see it largely as something negative, an indispensable evil. Social scientists and politicians alike try to pinpoint it, to limit it to certain areas of life, and to work out mechanisms to limit and control it. True, risk is also recognised as a part of success and achievement, as well as of pure excitement involved in testing fate and taking chances. In the West, risk is a source of anxiety, even if it can also be intoxicating and even addictive, as in increasingly risky sports and other leisure activities.

In Russia, the cultural attitude to risk is generally much more enthusiastic. This is expressed in the language by such sayings as 'He who does not take risks does not drink champagne' (*kto ne riskuiet, tot ne p'iet shampanskoie*), 'risk is a noble thing' (*risk – blagorodnoie delo*). Describing a person as a '*riskovyi paren*'', which corresponds to a disapproving English 'a fool-hardy guy', conveys, contrary to its English counterpart, a feeling of incredulous admiration; it amounts to admitting that a person who does not shrug off adventures other people would never dare to undertake, can harvest rewards far above the usual level.

I found that this attitude of inviting and welcoming risks was reflected in cultural behaviours that are difficult to explain by a conventional logic of the rational. For example, many foreigners I knew commented on the habit of Moscow car drivers to *pretend* to put on seatbelts, because traffic police could stop and fine a driver if he himself or his front-seat passengers did not have their seatbelts fastened. However, foreigners' attempts to *actually* buckle up their seatbelts have always caused the irritation and scorn of these same drivers. 'If you really end up in a crash, no seatbelts will save you', was the comment I often heard. In this case, neither the drivers nor their passengers would lose anything by following the rule that was in fact designed for their own safety, nor would they gain anything by refusing to follow it (other than perhaps a vague feeling of satisfaction that a Russian person usually feels when breaking a rule and getting away with it). As in many other cases, the logic of the logician here gives way to the logic of practice. According to this logic, the risk to be avoided is redefined as a challenge to fate, and the audacity of accepting its consequences.

The English word 'trust' is glossed by the Russian word '*doveriie*'. The latter, however, has a slightly different semantic domain from its English counterpart. The corresponding verb *doveriat'* applies mostly to close interpersonal relations of friends and kin, and refers to the transactions in private secrets rather than to money or social credibility. *Doveriie* also pertains to situations of entrusting someone with a valuable object or piece of property, like a car, an apartment, or a dear person, for temporary care: e.g. 'I entrust you with the care of [something/someone that is dear to me]'. In Russian, it is not natural to use trust/*doveriat'* to denote people's attitudes to their government or to a political leader; in this case the word used would be *verit'*, to have faith in, or *polagat'sia*, to rely on. In Russian Presidential election debates in the year 1999–2000, voters' trust in their candidates was denoted by the neologism *reiting* (from the English 'rating'), an indicator of popularity rather than trust. When Putin was elected president, and TV reporters interviewed people in the street, the comments were *my v nego verim* (we have faith in him), or *my emy verim* (we believe in him/in what he says). In business transactions, trust in one's partner would be rendered by *polagat'sia*, to rely on. To say that a person is trustworthy as a business companion, the adjective *nadezhnyi* would be used, translated as reliable, but stemming from the root *nadezhda*, hope. Generally, *doveriie* would be considered an overly personalised and emotional attitude to properly describe relations in the workplace or in business.

Luhmann makes an illuminating distinction between risk and danger (1993: 30). If a loss is attributed to a decision, if it is assessed as the consequence of a decision, we can speak of risk. If a loss is attributed to an environment, we speak of danger. This implies that when risk is involved, the person making the decision can somehow calculate the outcome, and thus foresee unfavourable consequences, at least to a degree. She can even avoid these consequences, for example, by deciding not to engage in a risky business. Risk is a factor of (at least partially) controlled environment. This is where the moment of responsibility, of the one who is exposed, comes in. When one risks and loses, one has only oneself to blame. In danger, if one is struck and hit, one is an unwitting victim, unfortunate but not guilty.

In the work of magi, we have seen how they consistently attempt to redefine the situations in which their clients find themselves as those of danger, rather than risk; danger caused by karma, destiny, their ancestors' immoral behaviour, or the lack of requisite channels. Thus understood, only the intervention of higher forces could bring things under any kind of appropriate control. Responsibility and accountability for persistent misfortune was lifted from the clients and shifted elsewhere, for example, to the sins of the forefathers, and, importantly, to the skills and endowments of the magus. This shift was not absolute, however. Thus, Katerina in her work with clients tried to make a distinction between 'karma' and their own foolishness, their stubbornness, their persistence in their own destructive patterns of attitude and behaviour. By making this distinction, and by persistently admonishing her clients to part with their 'illusions', she also tried to make them realise the limits of agency: hers, their own, and generally that of a human being. This was most striking in the cases of love magic, where her task, in the final analysis, was to bring home to clients that no magic can conjure up love, and that, 'if it was not meant', all magical means would only bond one person to another, in an unhealthy union. The notion of channels which are responsible for vocations and occupations served the same purpose: if a person did not have a money channel, she should not waste time engaging in business, and so on. The magus can remove the blocks to agency, take away the impediments to destiny, but she cannot change destiny itself or install new, previously nonexistent channels.

Keith Hart has spoken of trust as an expectation based on inconclusive evidence, tolerant of uncertainty and risk, and of confidence as a strong conviction based on substantial evidence. He went on to define hope as conviction without any evidence (1988: 187). It is this stubborn confidence without any substantial grounds, the ineradicable human faculty of hope, which sustains such people as described in this book, and helps them to rise again and continue with life after fending off the hardest blows.

Trusting expectation, which makes such a difference to decision making (Luhmann 1979: 25), is a learned attitude. It presupposes a structure and a history of social relationships that teaches individuals to 'trust trust', as Gambetta (1988) puts it. In a situation where the notion of trust is not applicable, there are other attitudes that can come in its stead. One is confidence in the self and in the power or charisma of the only helper – the powerful magus. As we have seen, one of the diacritics of power or charisma is this confidence *in spite of* uncertainty, when contingency is ruled out of the range of possibilities, as we have seen with Katerina. This confidence in her own power gives her clients in turn unswerving confidence in her and in themselves, allowing them to deal with frustrations and disappointments, interpreting them as omens, lessons to be learned or the consequences of someone else's omissions in the past. In addition to this there is the magus's strong '*mentál*,' her exceptional competence in the many fields of the game, coupled with the seeming lack of *illusio*, of visible investment in them. We have seen that this social competence, 'the feel for the game', for many games, is part of the charisma of human icons of power. Practical help is an important part of magical help; as a Russian (as well as an English) saying has it, two heads are better than one (*um khorosho, a dva luchshe*).

Like other human beings, people in Russia are driven by passions and desires; and like many other people in the world, they have to live with an uncertainty better described as danger. In conditions of life such as theirs, Bourdieu's rule-governed game often becomes gambling, Russian roulette, or, worse, a walk over a minefield. A player can leave the game if she chooses to; even a gambler can walk out of the gambling parlour provided her will is strong enough. A person walking a minefield does it because she has to – because her home and her children are on the other side. What drives a person walking the minefield? The need to reach the other side? Or can it be called desire? (And, as somebody has said, it is in the nature of desire to turn wishes into needs.) What magic in Russia does is to add to desire plus uncertainty the time dimension, to inform and support the attitude of hope. By investing all sorts of human ties with hope, from romantic passions to business transactions and the subordinations of the workplace, magi in Moscow make it possible for their clients to walk the minefield, and even sometimes to enjoy it. How is enjoyment possible in conditions of 'precarious presence', in what Bourdieu termed '*la misére du monde*'? There are many ways that people devise, and in Russia magic is one of them. It is about one main thing: the conjuring of hope.

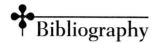

Bibliography

Abu-Lughod, Lila. 1991. 'Writing Against Culture'. In: *Recapturing Anthropology. Working in the Present*. R. Fox (ed.). Washington, DC: Washington University Press, pp.137–62.

Anderson, David. 2000. *Identity and Ecology in Arctic Siberia: the Number One Reindeer Brigade*. Oxford: Oxford University Press.

Asad, Talal. 2000. 'Agency and Pain: an Exploration'. *Culture and Religion*, 1(1): 29–60.

Balzer Mandelstam, Marjorie. 1993. 'Two Urban Shamans: Unmasking Leadership in Fin-de-Soviet Siberia'. In: *Perilous States: Conversations on Culture, Politics and Nation*. E. Marcus (ed.). Chicago, IL: University of Chicago Press, pp. 134–65.

———— 1999. *The Tenacity of Ethnicity: A Siberian Saga in Global Perspective*. Princeton, NJ: Princeton University Press.

Barker, Adelie (ed.) 1999. *Consuming Russia. Popular Culture, Sex, and Society Since Gorbachev*. Durham, NC: Duke University Press.

Beck, Ulrich. 1992. *The Risk Society*. Cambridge: Polity Press.

Belousova, Ekaterina. 2002. 'The Preservation of National Childbirth Traditions in the Russian Homebirth Community'. *The Journal of the Slavic and East European Folklore Association*, VII(2): 50–77. www.virginia.edu/~slavic/seefa/fall02.pdf

Berdahl, Daphne, Matti Bunzl and Martha Lampland (eds) 2000. *Altering States: Ethnographies of Transformation in Eastern Europe and in the Former Soviet Union*. Ann Arbor, MI: University of Michigan Press.

Berdyaev, Nikolai. 1990. *Istoki i smysl russkogo kommunizma*. Moskva: Nauka (Reprint from YMCA Press edition, Paris 1955). (*The Origin of Russian Communism*. Ann Arbor, MI: University of Michigan Press, 1972).

Birdsall, Karen. 2000. '"Everyday Crime" at the Workplace: Covert Earning Schemes in Russia's New Commercial Sector'. In: *Economic Crime in Russia*. A.V. Ledeneva and M. Kurchiyan (eds). The Hague: Kluwer Law International.

Bloch, Ernst. 1986. *The Principle of Hope*. Oxford: Basil Blackwell.

Bourdieu, Pierre. 1973. *Outline of a Theory of Practice*. Translated By R. Nice. Cambridge: Cambridge University Press.

———— 1990. *The Logic of Practice*. Stanford, CA: Polity Press.

———— 2000. *Pascalian Meditations*. Translated by Richard Nice. Cambridge: Polity Press.

Bourdieu, Pierre, and Loic J.D. Wacquant. 1992. *An Invitation to Reflexive Sociology*. Cambridge: Polity Press.

Bowie, Fiona. 2000. *The Anthropology of Religion. An Introduction.* Oxford and Massachussetts: Blackwell Publishers.

Boym, Svetlana. 1994. *Common Places. Mythologies of Everyday Life in Russia.* Cambridge and London: Harvard University Press.

Briggs, Jean. 1970. *Never In Anger. Portrait of an Eskimo Family.* Cambridge: Cambridge University Press.

Bruno, Martha. 1997. 'Women and Culture of Entrepreneurship'. In: *Post-Soviet Women: From Baltics to Central Asia.* M. Buckley (ed.). Cambridge: Cambridge University Press, pp. 56–74.

Caplan, Pat, Bell, D. and Karim W.J. (eds). 1993. *Gendered Fields: Women, Men, and Ethnography.* London: Routledge.

Chornyi, Vladimir. 2000. 'Russia: Multiple Financial System and Implications for Economic Crime'. In: *Economic Crime in Russia.* A.V. Ledeneva and M. Kurkchiyan (eds). The Hague: Kluwer Law International.

Coleman, Simon. 2000. *The Globalization of Charismatic Christianity.* Cambridge: Cambridge University Press.

Crick, Malcolm. 1992. 'Ali and Me. An Essay in Street-corner Anthropology'. In: *Anthropology and Autobiography.* J. Oakley and H. Callaway (eds). London: Routledge, pp.175–192.

Csordas, Thomas (ed.) 1994. *Embodiment and Experience.* Cambridge: Cambridge University Press.

——— 1997a. *Language, Charisma, and Creativity. The Ritual Life of a Religious Movement.* Berkeley, CA: University of California Press.

——— 1997b. *The Sacred Self. A Cultural Phenomenology of Religious Healing.* Berkeley, CA: University of California Press.

——— 2002. *Body/Meaning/Healing.* Houndmills and New York: Palgrave Macmillan.

Daniel, Valentine E. 1984. *Fluid Signs: Being a Person the Tamil Way.* Berkeley, CA: University of California Press.

——— 1994. 'The Individual in Terror'. In: *Embodiment and Experience: The Existential Ground of Culture and Self.* T. Csordas (ed.). Cambridge: Cambridge University Press.

Devisch, René. 1995. 'Frenzy, Violence, and Ethnical Renewal in Kinshasa'. *Public Culture,* 7(3): 593–629.

Droogers, André. 1994. *Syncretism, Power, Play.* Gothenburg: IASSA series.

Eco, Umberto. 1986. *A Theory of Semiotics.* Bloomington, IL: Indiana University Press.

Eisenstadt, S.N. (ed.) 1968. *Max Weber on Charisma and Institution Building.* Chicago, IL: University of Chicago Press.

Ekman, Paul. 1984. 'Expression and the Nature of Emotions'. In: *Approaches to Emotion.* K.R. Scherer and P. Ekman (eds). Hillsdale, NJ: Erlbaum.

Elgin, Catherine Z. 1996. 'Index and Icon Revisited'. In: *Peirce's Doctrine of Signs.* V. M. Colapietro and T.M. Olshevsky (eds). Berlin: Mouton de Gruyter.

Elliott, Anthony. 2002. *Psychoanalytic Theory: an Introduction.* Durham, NC: Duke University Press.

Evans-Prichard, E.E. 1976. *Witchcraft, Oracles, and Magic Among the Azande.* Oxford: Clarendon Press.

Foucault, Michel. 1980. *Power/Knowledge.* New York: Pantheon Books.

Frazer, James G. 1922. *The Golden Bough.* London: Macmillan.

Fromm, Erich. 1968. *The Revolution of Hope. Towards a Humanized Technology.* New York: Harper and Row.

Galeotti, Mark. 2000. 'The Russian Mafiya: Economic Penetration at Home and Abroad'. In: *Economic Crime in Russia.* A.V. Ledeneva and M. Kurkchiyan (eds). The Hague: Kluwer Law International Publishers.

Gambetta, Diego (ed.) 1998. *Trust. Making and Breaking Cooperative Relations.* Oxford: Blackwell.

Geertz, Clifford. 1977. 'Centers, Kings, and Charisma: Reflections of the Symbolics of Power'. In: *Culture and Its Creators: Essays in Honor of Edward Shils.* J. Ben-David and T.N. Clark (eds). Chicago, IL: University of Chicago Press, pp. 132–57.

Geshiere, Peter.1997. *The Modernity of Witchcraft. Politics and the Occult in Postcolonial Africa.* Charlottesville, VA: University Press of Virginia.

Glucklich, Ariel. 1997. *The End of Magic.* New York: Oxford Unversity Press.

Good, Byron. 1977. 'The Heart of What's the Matter. The Semantics of Illness in Iran'. *Culture, Medicine, and Psychiatry,* 1: 25–58.

———— 1994. *Medicine, Rationality, and Experience.* Cambridge: Cambridge University Press.

Grant, Bruce.1995. *In the Soviet House of Culture: a Century of Perestroikas.* Princeton, NJ: Princeton University Press.

Grant, Bruce and Nancy Ries. 2002. 'Foreword: The Shifting Fields of Culture and Society After Socialism'. In: *The Unmaking of Soviet Life. Everyday Economies After Socialism.* C. Humphrey (ed.). Ithaca, NY: Cornell University Press.

Grathoff, Richard H. 1970. *The Structure of Social Inconsistencies: A Contribution to a Unified Theory of Play, Game and Social Action.* The Hague: Martinus Nijhoff.

Greimas, Algirdas Julien and Jacques Fontanille.1993. *The Semiotics of Passions: From States of Affairs to States of Feelings.* Translated by Paul Perron and Frank Collins. Minneapolis, MN: University of Minnesota Press.

Hage, Ghassan. 2003. *Against Paarnoid Nationalism: Searching for Hope in a Shrinking Society.* Sydney: Pluto Press, London: Merlin Press.

Hammer, Olav. 1997. *På spaning efter helheten. New Age – en ny folktro?* Finland: Wahlström &Wikstrand.

Handelman, Don. 1990. *Models and Mirrors.* Cambridge: Cambridge University Press.

———— 1991. 'Symbolic Types, the Body, and Circus'. *Semiotica,* 85(3/4): 205–25.

———— n.d. *Microhistorical Anthropology: Towards a Prospective Perspective.*

Hann, Chris. 2002. 'Farewell to the Socialist "Other"'. In: *Postsocialism. Ideals, ideologies and Practices in Eurasia.* C.M. Hann (ed.). London and New York: Routledge.

Hannerz, Ulf. 1992. *Cultural Complexity. Studies in Social Organization of Meaning.* New York: Columbia University Press.

Hart, Keith. 1988. 'Kinship, Contract, and Trust: The Economic Organization of Migrants in an African City Slum'. In: *Trust. Making and Breaking Cooperative Relations.* D. Gambetta (ed.). Oxford: Blackwell, pp.176–93.

Humphrey, Caroline. 2002. *The Unmaking of Soviet Life. Everyday Economies After Socialism.* Ithaca, NY: Cornell University Press.

Innis, Robert. 1994. *Consciousness and the Play of Signs.* Bloomington, IL: Indiana University Press.

Ivanits, Linda J. 1989. *Russian Folk Belief.* Armonk, NY: Sharp.

Jackson, Michael. 2005. *Existential Anthropology.* Oxford and New York: Berghahn Books.

Kandiyoti, Deniz and Ruth Mandel (eds) 1998. *Market Reforms, Social Dislocations and Survival in Post-Soviet Central Asia.* Special issue of Central Asian Survey, 17(4).

Kapferer, Bruce. 1997. *The Feast of the Sorcerer.* Chicago and London: University of Chicago Press.

—— 2002. *Beyond Rationalism. Rethinking Magic, Witchcraft and Sorcery.* Oxford and New York: Berghahn Books.

Katz, Jack. 1999. *How Emotions Work.* Chicago, IL: University of Chicago Press.

Keane, Webb. 1997. *Signs of Recognition. Powers and Hazards of Representation in an Indonesian Society.* Berkeley, CA: University of California Press.

Kharitonova, V.I. 1994. *Portrety narodnykh tselitelei Rossii.* (The portraits of folk healers in Russia). Moskva: ENIOM.

—— 1995. *Traditsionnaia magiko-meditsinskaia praktika i sovremennoie narodnoie tselitel'stvo.* (Traditional magico-medical practice and contemporary folk healing). Etnologicheskii al'manakh. Russian Academy of Sciences, Miklukho-Maklai Institute of Ethnology and Anthropology.

—— 1999. 'Variatssii na temu … Stranstviia po miram Psikhicheskoi Vselennoi v traditsionnom i eksperientsial'nom shamanisme'. In: *'Izbranniki Dukhov'* – *'Izbravshiie dukhov'. Traditsionnoie shamanstvo i neoshamanizm* (Variations on the theme … Journeys in the worlds of Psychic Universe in traditional and experiential shamanism', In: 'Those chosen by Spirits – those who chose Spirits': Traditional Shamanism and Neoshamanism). Series 'Ethnological Studies of Shamanism and Other Traditional Beliefs and Practices', Moscow.

Kharkhordin, Oleg. 1999. *The Individual and the Collective in the Soviet Union.* Chicago, IL: University of Chicago Press.

Kleinman, Arthur. 1980. *Patients and Healers in the Context of Culture.* Berkeley, CA: University of California Press.

—— 1995. *Writing at the Margin. Discourse Between Anthropology and Medicine.* Berkeley, CA: University of California Press.

Kohut, Heinz. 1977. *The Restoration of the Self.* New York: International Universities Press.

Kuraiev, Andrei. 1998. *Okkultizm v Pravoslavii* (Occultism in the Russian Orthodoxy). Moskva: Blagovest.

Lambek, Michael and Jacqueline S. Solway. 2001. 'Just Anger: Scenarios of Indignation in Botswana and Madagascar'. *Ethnos,* 66(1): 49–72.

Langer, Susanne K. 1953. *Feeling and Form. A Theory of Art*. New York: Charles Scribner's Sons.

———— 1986 [1942]. 'Discursive and Presentational Forms'. In: *Semiotics: An Anthology*. R. Innis (ed.). Bloomington, IL: Indiana University Press.

Lash Scott and John Urry. 1994. *Economies of Signs and Space*. London: Sage Publications.

Leavitt, John. 1996. 'Meaning and Feeling in the Anthropology of Emotion'. *American Ethnologist* 23(3): 5114–539.

Ledeneva, Alena V. 1998. *Russia's Economy of Favors: Blat, Networking, and Informal Exchange*. Cambridge: Cambridge University Press.

Ledeneva, Alena V. and Marina Kurkchiyan (eds). 2000. *Economic Crime in Russia*. The Hague: Kluwer Law International.

Lévi-Strauss, Claude. 1963. 'The Effectiveness of Symbols'. In: *Structural Anthropology*. New York: Basic Books, pp. 167–85.

———— 1972. *Savage Mind*. London: Weidenfelt and Micolson.

Lindholm, Charles. 1990. *Charisma*. Oxford and Cambridge, CA: Blackwell.

———— 1995. 'Love as an Experience of Transcendence'. In: *Romantic Passion: A Universal Experience?* W. Jankowiak (ed.). New York: University of Columbia Press.

Lindquist, G. 2000a. 'Not My Will but Thine be Done: Church Versus Magic in Contemporary Russia'. *Culture and Religion*, 1(2): 247–76.

———— 2000b. 'In Search of the Magic Flow: Magic and Market in Contemporary Russia'. *Urban Anthropology*, 29(4): pp. 315–57.

———— 2001a. 'The Culture of Charisma'. *Anthropology Today*, 17(2): 3–8.

———— 2001b. 'Gurus, Wizards and Energo-information fields: Alternative Medicine in Post-Communist Russia'. *The Anthropology of East Europe Review*, 19(1): 16–28.

———— 2001c. 'Transforming Signs: Typologies of Affliction in Contemporary Russian Magic and Healing'. *Ethnos*, 66(2): 181–206.

———— 2001d. 'Breaking the Waves: Voodoo Magic in the Russian Cultural Ecumene'. In: R. Stryker and J. Patico (eds) *The Paradoxes of Progress: Globalization and Postsocialist Cultures. Kroeber Anthropological Society Papers*, 86: 93–112.

———— 2002a. 'Spirits and Souls of Business: New Russians, Magic and the Esthetics of Kitsch'. *Journal of Material Culture*, 7(3): 329–43.

———— 2002b. 'Healing Efficacy and the Construction of Charisma: a Family's Journey Through the Multiple Medical Field in Russia'. *Anthropology and Medicine*. 9(3): 337–58.

Luhmann, Niklas. 1979. *Trust and Power*. New York: John Wiley and Sons.

———— 1988. 'Familiarity, Confidence, Trust: Problems and Alternatives'. In: *Trust. Making and Breaking Cooperative Relations*. D. Gambetta (ed.). Oxford: Blackwell.

———— 1993. *Risk: A Sociological Theory*. Translated by Rhodes Barret. The Haague: Aldine de Gruyter.

Luhrmann, Tanya. 1989. *Persuasions of the Witch's Craft. Ritual Magic in Contemporary England*. Oxford: Blackwell.

Lupton, Deborah. 1998. *The Emotional Self: A Sociocultural Exploration*. London: Sage.

Lyon, M.L. and J.M. Barbalet. 1994. 'Society's Body: Emotion and the Somatization of Social Theory'. In: *Embodiment and Experience*. T. Csordas (ed.). Cambridge: Cambridge University Press, pp. 48–68.

MacCormack, Carol. 1981. 'Health Care and the Concept of Legitimacy'. *Social Science and Medicine*, 15B: 423–28.

―――― 1986. 'The Articulation of Western and Traditional Systems of Health Care'. In: *The Professionalization of African Medicine*. G.L. Chavunduka and M. Last (eds). Manchester: Manchester University Press.

Malinowski, Bronislaw. 1922. *Argonauts of the Western Pacific: an Account of Native Enterprise and Adventure in the Archipelagoes of Melanesian New Guinea*. London: Routledge and Kegan Paul.

―――― 1948. *Magic, Science, and Religion, and other essays*. Boston, MA: Beacon.

―――― 1965. *Coral Gardens and their Magic*. Bloomington, IL: Indiana University Press.

Mauss, Marcel. 1972. *A General Theory of Magic*. Translated by Robert Brain. London: Routledge.

Meshcherkina, Elena. 2002. *Bytiie muzhskogo soznaniia: Opyt rekonstruktsii maskulinnoi identichnosti crednego I rabochego klassa*. (The being of male consciousness: Reconstruction of masculine identities of the middle and working class). In: *O muzhe(n)stvennosti (On Masculinity)*. S. Oushakine (ed.). Moscow: *Novoie literaturnoie obozreniie*, pp. 268–87.

Milton, Kay. 2002. *Loving Nature. Towards an Ecology of Emotions*. London and New York: Routledge.

Myers, Fred. 1998. 'The Logic and Meaning of Anger Among Pintupi Aborigines'. *Man* (NS), 23: 589–610.

Nagengast, Carole. 1991. *Reluctant Socialists, Rural Entrepreneurs, Class Culture, and the Polish State*. Boulder, CO: Westview.

Narayan, Kirin. 1993. 'How Native is a 'Native' Anthropologist?' *American Anthropologist*, 95: 671–686.

Oushakine, Sergei. 2000. 'In the State of Post-Soviet Aphasia: Symbolic Development in Contemporary Russia'. *Europe-Asia Studies*. 52(6): 991–1016.

Pachenkov, Oleg. 2001. 'Ratsional'noie "zakoldovyvaniie mira": sovremennyie rossiiskiie "magi"'. (Rational 'reenchantment of the world': the contemporary 'magi' in Russia). In: *Nevidimyie grani sotsial'noi real'nosti. (The unseen facets of social reality)* V.9. St.Petersburg: Center for Independent Social Research. pp. 96–109.

Peirce, Charles Sanders. 1932. Collected Papers. V. 1–6, C. Hartshorne and P. Weiss (eds). Cambridge, MA: Harvard University Press.

―――― 1958. Collected Papers. V. 7–8. A. Burks (ed.). Cambridge, MA: Harvard University Press.

Peirce, Charles Sanders and Victoria Lady Welby. 1977. *Semiotics and Significs: The Correspondence Between Charles S. Peirce and Victoria Lady Welby*. C.S. Hadwick (ed.). Bloomington, IL: Indiana University Press.

—— 1985. 'Logic as Semiotic: the Theory of Signs'. In: *Semiotics: An Introductory Anthology*. R. Innis (ed.). Bloomington, IL: Indiana University Press.

Perron, Paul and Paolo Fabbri. 1993. 'Foreword'. In: A. Greimas and J. Fontanille (eds). *The Semiotics of Passions. From States of Affairs to States of Feelings*. Minneapolis, MS: University of Minnesota Press.

Pesmen, Dale. 2000. *Russia and Soul: An Exploration*. Ithaca, NY: Cornell University Press.

Petryna, Ariadna. 2002. *Life Exposed: Biological Citizens After Chernobyl*. Princeton, NJ: Princeton University Press.

Rancour-Laferriere, Daniel. 1995. *The Slave Soul of Russia. Moral Masochism and the Cult of Suffering*. New York and London: New York University Press.

Rappaport, Roy. 1999. *Ritual and Religion in the Making of Humanity*. Cambridge: Cambridge University Press.

Ries, Nancy. 1997. *Russian Talk. Culture and Conversation During Perestroika*. Ithaca, NY: Cornell University Press.

Ries, Nancy. 2002. ' "Honest Bandits" and "Warped People": Russian Narratives about Money, Corruption, and Moral Decay'. In: *Ethnography in Unstable Places. Everyday Lives in Contexts of Dramatic Political Change*. C.J. Greenhouse, E. Mertz and K.B. Warren (eds). Durham, NC: Duke University Press.

Rivkin-Fish, Michele. 1999. 'Sexuality Education in Russia: Defining Pleasure and Danger for a Fledgling Democratic Society'. *Social Science and Medicine*, 49: 801–14.

Rodriguez Laretta, Enrique. 2002. *'Gold Is Illusion'. The Garimpeiros of Tapajos Valley in the Brazilian Amazonia*. Stockholm Studies in Social Anthropology, Stockholm: Sweden.

Ryan, W.F. 1999. *The Bathhouse at Midnight. Magic in Russia*. University Park, PA: Pennsylvania State University Press.

Sacks, Oliver. 1995. *An Anthropologist on Mars*. London: Picador.

Samosiuk I.Z. and Lyseniuk V.P. 1994. *Metod Fol'ia*. Kiev.

Sartre, Jean Paul. 1976. *The Emotions: Outline of a Theory*. Translated by B. Frechtman. New York: Philosophical Library.

Seabright, Paul. (ed.) 2000. *The Vanishing Ruble: Barter Networks and Non-Monetary Transactions in Post-Soviet Societies*. Cambridge: Cambridge University Press.

Sergeyev, Victor. 1998. *The Wild East. Crime and Lawlessness in Post-Communist Russia*. Armonk, London: M.E. Sharpe.

Shils, E. 1968. 'Charisma'. In: *International Encyclopedia of the Social Sciences*, vol. 2. D.E. Shils (ed.). New York: Macmillan.

Shlapentokh, Vladimir. 1989. *Public and Private Life of the Soviet People. Changing Values in Post-Stalinist Russia*. New York: Oxford University Press.

Singer, Milton. 1978. 'For a Semiotic Anthropology'. In *Sight, Sound, and Sense*. T.A. Sebeok (ed.). Bloomington, IL: Indiana University Press.

—— 1980. 'Signs of the Self: An Exploration in Semiotic Anthropology'. *American Anthropologist*, 82(3): 485–507.

Skorupski, John. 1976. *Symbol and Theory: A Philosophical Study of Theories of Religion in Social Anthropology.* Cambridge: Cambridge University Press.

Skultans, Vieda. 1998. *The Testimony of Lives.* London and New York: Routledge.

Stephen, Michele. 1995. *A'aisa's Gift. A Study of Magic and the Self.* Berkeley, CA: University of California Press.

Tambiah, Stanley J. 1968. 'The Magical Power of Words'. *Man* (NS), 3(2): 175–208.

———— 1985. 'The Sources of Charismatic Leadership: Max Weber Revisited'. In: *Comparative Social Dynamics.* E. Cohen, M. Lissak and U. Almagor (eds). Boulder, CO: Westview Press, pp. 73–81.

———— 1990. *Magic, Science, Religion, and the Scope of Rationality.* Cambridge: Cambridge University Press.

Taussig, Michael. 1987. *Shamanism, Colonialism, and the White Man. A Study in Terror and Healing.* Chicago, IL: University of Chicago Press.

———— 1993. *Mimesis and Alterity.* New York and London: Routledge.

Verdery, Katherine. 1996. *What is Socialism, and What Comes Next?* Princeton, NJ: Princeton University Press.

Vitebski, Piers. 1995. 'From Cosmology to Environmentalism: Shamanism as Local Knowledge in a Global Setting'. In: *Counterworks: Managing the Diversity of Knowledge.* R. Fardon (ed.). London and New York: Routledge, pp. 182–203.

Volkov, Vadim. 2000. 'Organized Violence, Market Building, and State Formation in Post-Communist Russia'. In: *Economic Crime in Russia.* A.V. Ledeneva and M. Kurkchiyan (eds). The Hague: Kluwer Law International Publishers.

Weber, Max. 1970. *Essays in Sociology.* Translated by H.H. Gerth and C. Wright Mills. London: Routledge and Kegan Paul.

———— 1964. *The Theory of Social and Economic Organization.* New York: Free Press.

Whittaker, Elvi. 1992. 'The Birth of the Anthropological Self and its Career'. *Ethos* 20: 191–219.

Whyte, Susan. 1998. *Questioning Misfortune. The Pragmatics of Uncertainty in Eastern Uganda.* Cambridge: Cambridge University Press.

Wierzbicka, Anna. 1994. 'Emotion, Language, and Cultural Scripts'. In: *Emotion and Culture: Empirical Studies of Mutual Influence.* S. Kitayama and R. Markus (eds). Washington DC: American Psychological Association, pp.133–96.

Winnicott, D.W. 1958. 'Primary Maternal Preoccupations'. In: *Through Pediatrics to Psychoanalysis.* London: Hogarth Press.

Wolman, Benjamin. (ed.). 1996. *The Encyclopedia of Psychiatry, Psychology, and Psychoanalysis.* New York: Henry Holt.

Yurchak, Aleksei. 2002. 'Muzhskaia ekonomika: "Ne do glupostei, kogda karieru kuiesh"'(Masculine economy.) In: *O muzhe(n)stvennosti* (On Masculinity). S. Oushakine (ed.). Moscow: Novoie literaturnoie obozreniie, pp. 245–66.

Zaner, Richard M. 1981. *The Context of Self: A Phenomenological Inquiry Using Medicine as a Clue.* Athens, OH: Ohio University Press.

Index

A

Abu-Lughod, Lila, xi, xvii
affect, xi, 21, 83, 85–86
  grammar of, 2, 121, 172
  logic of, 5
affliction, 55, 58, 63, 65–66, 68, 70, 80, 83, 103
  terms of, 13, 50, 53, 56, 69, 70–73, 172, 195, 209
  typology of, 54
agency, 3, 4, 7–8, 13, 16, 18, 63, 74, 90, 94, 97, 106, 108–110, 124, 128, 133, 149–50, 156–7, 168, 189, 190, 192, 199, 208, 225, 229, 235
  channels of, xviii, 2, 8, 10, 126
  and friendship, 208
  and hope, 8
  limits of, 185, 234
alterity, legitimation by, 39
AMSAD (computer diagnostics), 35, 143
Anderson, David, 1
anger, 55, 83, 90–94, 107–110, 150, 156, 181, 185–87, 191, 203
  semiosis of, 91, 108
aphasia, post-Soviet, xv, 20, 74, 87
archetypes, 138
Asad, Talal, 7
asceticism, 128

B

babka (*babushka*), 28–29, 31, 33, 161

Balzer, Marjorie, 22n.1, 52n.2
Barbalet, J.M., 84
Barker, Adelie, 1
barter, 125, 200
Beck, Ulrick, 210
Being, augmentation of, 21. *See also conatus*
  phenomenology of, 5–6, 8
belief, 1, 9, 24, 36, 52n.2, 55–56, 66, 171, 208
belonging, 20
Belousova, Ekaterina, 29
Berdahl, Daphne, 1
Berdyaev, Nikolai, 168
Birdsall, Karen, 50
blat, 125–27, 205–6, 208, 227n.1
Bloch, Ernest, 6
Bourdieu, Pierre, 4–6, 9–10, 12, 21, 172, 185, 228, 230–31, 236
Bowie, Fiona, 55
Boym, Svetlana, xv, xvi, 63, 111, 165
bribe, 15, 97, 123, 125, 147, 206, 219, 223, 232
Briggs, Jean, 93
bureaucracy, x, 3, 142, 146, 185
business schemes, 216–18

C

Caplan, Pat, 116
Carnegie, Dale, 206
charisma, xviii, xx, 20, 36–37, 94, 114–15, 127, 129, 133, 137, 145, 157, 163, 165, 181, 214, 235
  bond of, 116, 133